Register Now for Online Access to You...

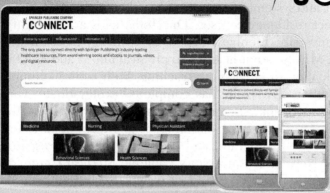

COMPANY

Your print purchase of *Practice-Based Scholarly Inquiry and the DNP Project, 2e,* **includes online access to the contents of your book**—increasing accessibility, portability, and searchability!

Access today at:

http://connect.springerpub.com/content/book/978-0-8261-3494-3 or scan the QR code at the right with your smartphone and enter the access code below.

B2WV99XR

Scan here for quick access.

SPRINGER / PUBLISHING COMPANY

View all our products at springerpub.com

Cheryl Holly, EdD, RN, ANEF, FNAP, is professor, senior methodologist, and codirector of the Northeast Institute for Evidence Synthesis and Translation (NEST) at Rutgers School of Nursing, an inaugural Joanna Briggs Institute Center of Excellence. Dr. Holly holds a joint faculty appointment in the School of Nursing and the School of Public Health. She teaches DNP program courses in population health, implementation science, and systematic review, and works with DNP students during their project residency courses. Dr. Holly holds a BS in nursing from Pace University, Lienhard School of Nursing, Pleasantville, New York, and an MEd in adult health and physical illness and EdD in research and evaluation in curriculum/teaching, both from Columbia University. In addition, Dr. Holly has completed postgraduate work in comprehensive meta-analysis and advanced meta-analysis at the Statistics Institute. Dr. Holly has been an associate dean, department chair, director of a DNP program, and director of nursing research and informatics at New York University's Langone Medical Center in New York City, and a senior vice president of quality clinical resource management. She is certified as a train-the-trainer in comprehensive systematic review by the Joanna Briggs Institute and has offered workshops on comprehensive systematic review across the country. Dr. Holly is the coordinator of the Eastern Nursing Research Society's Research Interest Group on Comprehensive Systematic Review and Knowledge Translation, and she is a member of the Committee of Directors of the Joanna Briggs Institute of Nursing and Midwifery, the Evidence Translation Group, the Cochrane Nursing Care Field, the Cochrane Injuries Group, and the Joanna Briggs Institute Scientific Methodology Group on Umbrella Reviews and Rapid Reviews. She is also a member of the Patient-Centered Outcomes Research Institute (PCORI) Advisory Board on Health Disparities and Health Delivery Systems. She serves as manuscript reviewer for several journals, including *Nursing Outlook*, *Nursing Education Perspectives*, the *American Journal of Nursing*, and the *International Journal of Evidence-Based Healthcare*. She is a founding member of the Implementation Science and Synthesis Network of the Americas. Dr. Holly has been principal investigator (PI), co-PI, or project director of several funded research projects. She has published extensively and presented nationally and internationally in the areas of evidence-based practice, systematic review, and knowledge translation and critical care nursing, and she has won awards for some of this work. Dr. Holly is a fellow in the Academy of Nursing Education, a distinguished scholar and fellow of the National Academies of Practice, and a clinical fellow of the Joanna Briggs Institute.

Practice-Based Scholarly Inquiry and the DNP Project

Second Edition

CHERYL HOLLY, EdD, RN, ANEF, FNAP

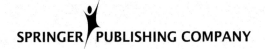

SPRINGER PUBLISHING COMPANY

Springer Publishing Company, LLC
11 West 42nd Street
New York, NY 10036
www.springerpub.com
http://connect.springerpub.com

Acquisitions Editor: Margaret Zuccarini
Compositor: Amnet Systems

ISBN: 978-0-8261-3493-6
ebook ISBN: 978-0-8261-3494-3
Instructor's PowerPoints ISBN: 978-0-8261-3495-0
DOI: 10.1891/9780826134943

Instructors Materials: Qualified instructors may request supplements by emailing textbook@springerpub.com.

19 20 21 22 23 / 5 4 3 2 1

The author and the publisher of this Work have made every effort to use sources believed to be reliable to provide information that is accurate and compatible with the standards generally accepted at the time of publication. Because medical science is continually advancing, our knowledge base continues to expand. Therefore, as new information becomes available, changes in procedures become necessary. We recommend that the reader always consult current research and specific institutional policies before performing any clinical procedure. The author and publisher shall not be liable for any special, consequential, or exemplary damages resulting, in whole or in part, from the readers' use of, or reliance on, the information contained in this book. The publisher has no responsibility for the persistence or accuracy of URLs for external or third-party Internet websites referred to in this publication and does not guarantee that any content on such websites is, or will remain, accurate or appropriate.

Library of Congress Cataloging-in-Publication Data

Names: Holly, Cheryl, author.
Title: Practice-based scholarly inquiry and the DNP project / Cheryl Holly.
Other titles: Preceded by (work): Scholarly inquiry and the DNP capstone.
Description: Second edition. | New York, NY : Springer Publishing Company,
    LLC, [2019] | Preceded by Scholarly inquiry and the DNP capstone / [edited
    by] Cheryl Holly. | Includes bibliographical references and index.
Identifiers: LCCN 2018058341 (print) | LCCN 2018059928 (ebook) | ISBN
    9780826134943 (eBook) | ISBN 9780826134936 (print : alk. paper) | ISBN
    9780826134950 (instructor's powerpoints) | ISBN 9780826134943 (e-book)
Subjects: | MESH: Clinical Nursing Research—methods | Research Design |
    Advanced Practice Nursing
Classification: LCC RT81.5 (ebook) | LCC RT81.5 (print) | NLM WY 20.5 | DDC
    610.73072—dc23
LC record available at https://lccn.loc.gov/2018058341

Contact us to receive discount rates on bulk purchases.
We can also customize our books to meet your needs.
For more information please contact sales@springerpub.com

Printed in the United States of America.

Contents

Preface

Advanced practice nurses study long and hard to achieve the skills and knowledge necessary to provide safe and cost-effective patient-centered care across a variety of practice settings. As experts in a practice discipline, advanced practice nurses are practice scholars. This book is intended to support that scholarship. It is written for advanced practice nurses, students in advanced practice nursing programs, and doctoral students interested in conducting clinically based projects. Faculty may also benefit from this book. The content selected reflects my work with doctor of nursing practice (DNP) students over 14 years.

The book is presented in two sections, and is wholly devoted to DNP scholarly practice and the DNP project. The first section concerns scholarship. Chapter 1 is about being a scholar and engaging in scholarly inquiry. It is written with the understanding that there are complex relationships involving practice and clinical wisdom. Reflection allows knowledge to grow from practice. It is practice that provides an avenue for scholarly practice and, therefore, inquiry. Chapter 2 is about scholarly inquiry and the domains of scholarship: application, discovery, integration, and teaching. Chapters 3 and 4 are new to the second edition. Chapter 3 describes the DNP project. As a scholar, the DNP student completes a final scholarly project, most commonly called a *DNP capstone project*, although many other names are also used. These projects reflect the mastery of the discipline acquired during doctoral education and demonstrate the necessary engagement for practice—scholarship that will influence healthcare outcomes in the practice setting. Chapter 4 is about searching the literature for evidence to support a project and critically appraising that literature. These are both important skills for a scholar-practitioner and important steps in a successful DNP project.

The second section concerns the methods of scholarly inquiry that lend themselves to clinical projects. Chapter 5 introduces action research, a reflective process that is grounded in context and investigates real-world situations. It is a constantly evolving method of inquiry conducted within familiar settings by teams working together for the resolution of practice problems. Chapter 6 details how to construct a case study. A case study allows investigation into a clinical problem within a context bounded by time, place, and activity, in which multiple sources of evidence are used. Chapter 7 is about qualitative descriptive projects. A qualitative descriptive method involves a direct description of events using the terms provided by the subject. Chapter 8 is about clinical interventional projects. Because nursing is a practice discipline, an understanding of how particular interventions work and in what context they work can inform practice and improve patient care. Chapter 9 is about systematic review, the findings of which are used by practitioners to make point-of-care decisions based on the best available evidence for a focused clinical question. Chapter 10 describes integrative review. An integrative review project takes a traditional review of the literature one step further by providing a more substantial contribution to knowledge using a transparent process and by providing a critical appraisal of the literature used in the review. Chapter 11 explores quality improvement, the focus of which is on systems and processes that can be improved. Chapter 12 is about program evaluation, which is the process of collecting, analyzing, and using data to measure the impact or outcomes of a program or project. Chapters 13 and 14 are new to this edition. Chapter 13 describes descriptive observational projects within the framework of time, place, and person. Chapter 14 is about disseminating the findings of the DNP project.

Advance practice nurses can develop clinically focused practice projects that not only advance nursing practice but also inform the redesign of healthcare considering new and emerging healthcare mandates. The aim of the second edition is to provide a foundation to accomplish this goal and disseminate the results.

Cheryl Holly
Sandy Hook, Connecticut

Qualified instructors may obtain access to PowerPoints by emailing textbook@springerpub.com.

Part I

CHAPTER 1

The DNP and Scholarly Practice

■ OBJECTIVES

At the end of this chapter, you will be able to:

- Define scholarship.
- Explain the nature of professional practice.
- Describe the contribution of scholarship to professional practice.
- Describe strategies to support interprofessional collaboration.
- Develop a plan for scholarly practice.

■ KEY CONCEPTS

- Scholarship is an intentional activity shaped by experience and meaning.
- Experienced practitioners have the capacity to adapt to the complex phenomenological aspects of practice.
- A wise clinical nurse can make accurate choices and act without knowing in advance exactly what the consequences will be.
- A reflective practitioner is one who learns both from experience and about experience.
- Inherent in wisdom is the understanding that interprofessional collaboration is necessary for optimal patient outcomes.
- A wise scholar in a practice discipline is a reflective practitioner able to engage in interprofessional collaboration that advances the teaching, research, practice, and policies of nursing practice through orderly and regular inquiry.

INTRODUCTION

Scholarship refers to a set of practices used by scholars to make claims about the world that are as valid and reliable as possible. Inherent in this set of practices is the requirement that claims made are disseminated to the public and the profession. Scholarship embodies methods that advance the teaching, research, practice, and guiding policies of an academic field of study through systematic inquiry. Scholarship activities are noted by their significance to a specific profession or discipline, are creative, are documented, provide the essential information necessary to be replicated or extended, and are peer reviewed (American Association of Colleges of Nursing [AACN], 2017).

Scholars use the scientific method to investigate phenomena, acquire new knowledge, or transfer knowledge. The scientific method is a process by which scholars attempt to build an accurate representation of the world. To be termed *scientific*, a method of inquiry must be based on gathering observable, empirical, and measurable evidence subject to specific principles of reasoning. The basic steps in the scientific method are:

- Ask a question.
- Search the literature.
- Construct a hypothesis.
- Test the hypothesis.
- Collect and analyze data.
- Draw a conclusion.
- Report and disseminate results.

A scholar can also seek to gain an in-depth understanding of the social world through qualitative research. The aim of qualitative research is to understand the meanings, practices, behaviors, and processes of human experience (Benner, 1994). A naturalistic approach is used to observe participants—individuals, groups, communities, or a given culture—in their natural environment in an attempt to understand phenomena within a real context, the context within which they occur, without any attempt to manipulate or test the phenomenon of interest (Bradley, Curry, & Devers, 2007).

Being a scholar and engaging in scholarly inquiry in a practice discipline, such as nursing, requires an understanding of the nature of practice. Although scientific practices predominate in most settings, there are contextual issues that may require a different approach. According to Pearson (2011), "expert nurses possess deep sensitivity to the social, cultural, and biological contexts of their patients, and an ability to adapt rapidly to the unpredictable day-to-day dynamics of the hospital, clinic or community" (p. 443). In other words, the nature of nursing practice is more than the concepts propagated by curricula and standards. Nursing practice is an intellectually and emotionally challenging endeavor, often requiring quick judgments and rapid responses to life-threatening conditions where little margin for error exists. It is essential for nursing practice scholars to keep this in mind as they inquire into the nature of nursing practice.

One's practice is personal, based on his or her experiences. Experienced practitioners have the capacity to adapt to the complex phenomenological aspects of practice. Intuition may play a role in this adaptation, as Schraeder and Fischer (1986) have commented that "intuitive perception in nursing practice is the ability to experience the elements of a clinical situation as a whole, to solve a problem or reach a decision with limited concrete information" (p. 161). In other words, there is a "gut feeling" or sixth sense at work without benefit of analysis. According to Ruth-Sahd (2003), intuition is a key element in discovery, holistic problem solving, understanding, and knowledge generation. Dossey, Keegan, and Guzzetta (2003) identify six characteristics of nursing intuition:

■ Pattern recognition—the ability to put things together given disparate pieces
■ Similarity recognition—the ability to see resemblances and compare them
■ Common sense and understanding
■ Skilled know-how
■ A sense of salience—knowing what is right and most important
■ Deliberate rationality—the ability to think about things with a purpose in mind

Intuition is often combined with analysis, particularly in situations that are familiar. In a study of novice clinicians, Price (2004) reported that although most participants relied more heavily on analysis than on intuition, use of intuition when faced with familiar complications of care was associated with more accurate decision-making, particularly in guiding attention to relevant cues. Further, when any new complication arose, use of intuition appeared to hamper decision-making, particularly for those in an observer role. In an older study of nurses' intuition, Rew and Barrow (1987) concluded that nurses reflect on the meaning and consequences of acting on limited information, which both mitigates the linear approach of the medical model and enhances nursing practice.

This chapter focuses on the nature of nursing practice in a real-world context—a discussion to which clinical wisdom and reflective practice contribute—in which intuition, knowledge, and skill are over-arching components and in which scholarly inquiry into that practice is both appreciated and required.

CHARACTERISTICS OF PRACTICE

A practice implies that actions take "place in particular situations at particular times with particular persons within a complex set of contingencies that affect practitioners, service users, their interpretations and meanings, and how they engage with each other" (Gilgun, 2010, p. 10). In other words, individuals are embedded in events and attribute meaning to each of these events, and based on these meanings, they practice.

Practice, however, is not just an activity; rather it involves intentional action and draws on disciplinary knowledge, personal knowledge, and technical knowledge (Kemmis, 2009). *Disciplinary knowledge* encompasses knowledge in existing frameworks and theories related to a specific discipline or area of practice, each with its own language and specified concepts. These theories and frameworks explicate the landscape of each discipline. Nursing by its very nature is multidisciplinary, as its major concern is the biopsychosocial–spiritual human in interaction with the environment (Parse, 1999). *Personal knowledge* is knowledge possessed by any individual gained through cultural experiences, observation, or personal experiences. It is unique to each individual. *Technical knowledge* is the acquisition of skills required for a practice discipline. In other words, practice is shaped by experience, is culturally located, and employs learned competencies and skills (Kemmis, 2009). Practice involves real-world and critical reasoning about how to act in given situations, which allows development of a professional role. Carper's (1978) classic four fundamental ways of knowing have been used as a framework for practitioner development. These are: empirical knowing, aesthetic knowing, ethical knowing, and personal knowing (Table 1.1). According to Carper, "there is a need to examine the kinds of knowing that provide the discipline with its particular perspectives and significance. An understanding of the four fundamental patterns of knowing makes possible an increased awareness of the complexity and diversity of nursing knowledge" (p. 21). Understanding the complex interplay among these four patterns allows exploration of the various concepts linked to nursing's educational, evaluative, and practice processes (Zander, 2007). In illustration, Zander (2007) relates this story from her time working in the Marshall Islands with a group of nursing students from the United States:

TABLE 1.1

NURSING WAYS OF KNOWING

Way or Pattern of Knowing	Foundation	Characteristics	Example of a Question for Inquiry
Empirical	Science Theories Models Principles	Objective Verifiable	What is the effect of noise on blood pressure? What components of a multicomponent approach to delirium work best for prevention?
Aesthetic	Art Skill Experience	Intangible Individual	What is the meaning of "advanced nursing practice" to those who practice it? What is the value of certification to the bedside nurse?
Ethical	Morality Philosophy Personal values	Rights Duty	What moral principles are evident in nurses' decisions regarding end-of-life care? How do nurses handle difficult moral situations?
Personal	Authenticity	Awareness of self Interpersonal relationships Engagement	How do nurses describe their role in patient situations when the patient lacks autonomy? What is the impact of patient and family engagement on nursing practice?

Source: Carper, B. A. (1978). Fundamental patterns of knowing in nursing. *Advances in Nursing Science, 1*(1), 13–23. doi:10.1097/00012272-197810000-00004; Zander, P. (2007). Ways of knowing in nursing: The historical evolution of a concept. *Journal of Theory Construction and Testing, 11*(1), 6–11.

A Marshallese man from one of the outer islands had been brought to the hospital for an emergency below the knee amputation of his right leg. He was septic and for the first few days existed on intravenous (IV) fluids. After his condition improved from very critical to critical, he demanded that the IV be removed. The patient's doctor ordered Gatorade to replace the fluids and electrolytes formerly provided by the IV. The patient refused to drink it. Upon informing the author of their patient's refusal to drink the Gatorade, the students were instructed to ask the man's wife to give him some water from the coconuts she had in the room (*aesthetics*). The students were shocked and asked for rationale for this direction. During a prior experience in the Marshall Islands the author had been told about coconut water being used during the Second World War when no IV fluids were available (*empirics*). After this episode, a special relationship or bond developed between the Marshallese man, who wanted to be in charge of his situation, and the author, who he allowed to take charge when necessary (*personal*). (p. 10, italics added)

These patterns are also seen in several studies on the characteristics of professional nursing practice. Girard, Linton, and Besner (2005), for example, found that collaboration was the most prominent characteristic of practice and that professional nursing practice means

working in partnership with other nurses and health professionals in providing client care, being highly organized in managing activities and time, having the ability to manage many complex tasks simultaneously, working autonomously as appropriate and having an open mind and nonjudgmental manner. (para 9)

Competence and commitment were also seen as important components of a professional practice model.

A professional practice evolves, and to practice professionally requires constant learning. In a qualitative study of the meaning of scholarly practice, Riley and Beal (2013) found that in a study of nurses, practice development followed a pattern of recognition that practice is a journey that goes from being timid and unknowing to recognizing personal learning needs in which the nurses sought situations in which they needed greater knowledge and experience. Finally came the realization that patients assisted nurses in their practice development. The need to answer patients' and families' questions required the nurses to simplify complex information for both their own and patients' learning. They explained that although patients saw them as caregivers, not learners, nurses saw themselves as learners on a journey toward being knowledgeable, comfortable, confident, and skilled practitioners.

Clinical Wisdom

Being wise implies that one is shrewd, intelligent, astute, and clever. Confucius (551–479 BCE) wrote, "By three methods we may learn wisdom: first, by reflection, which is noble; second, by imitation, which is easiest; and third by experience, which is the most bitter." Clinical wisdom is about knowledge, experience, empathy, integrity, resourcefulness, and inspiration. Benner, Hooper-Kyriakidis, and Stannard (2011) posited that clinical wisdom is based on clinical judgment and a thinking-in-action approach that encompasses feelings, emotions, and senses with the acceptance that there is an intellectual process and knowledge base made visible through actions and deeds. The distinctive features of wisdom include recognition of contextual factors and the place of each person in a situation (McKie et al., 2012). In other words, clinically wise nurses have the ability to connect theoretical physiological signs with patient presentation and find or develop the resources necessary to ensure optimal patient outcome. They are able to respond quickly and appropriately to patient events. Clinically wise nurses act on behalf of patients who are unable to act for themselves, prevent crises, and assume clinical leadership as needed (Seiden, 2010). The wise nurse who achieves wisdom is tolerant of diversity and differences. For example, in a study of Danish nurses, Uhrenfeldt and Hall (2007) found that clinically wise nurses made decisions based on changes in patients' condition. Assessing situations was connected to the nurses' thinking and ethical discernment, transparency about actions taken, and setting mutual goals with patients. Calmness, assessment of situations, and focusing on patient responses were essential to decision-making. The researchers noted that unhealthy working conditions served as a barrier, which may lead the wise nurse back to nonproficient performance, threatening her or his ability to think and act with responsibility. An unhealthy work environment is one in which people feel unvalued and underappreciated. This can range from bullying, screaming, and being talked down to, to more subtle forms of poor communication, setting people up for failure, mismanagement, and environment of hostility. It can come from your supervisors, peers, or patients. Establishing and sustaining healthy work environments must be a priority for nurses to make optimal contributions in caring for patients and patients' families. The ingredients necessary for a healthy work environment are skilled communication, true collaboration, effective decision-making, appropriate staffing, meaningful recognition, and authentic leadership (American Association of Critical-Care Nurses [AACN], 2016).

Inherent in being wise is understanding that these ingredients must be aligned with collaboration. Collaboration involves a process of cooperation and teamwork centered on mutual goals. The act of collaborating is usually considered a necessary component of success among individuals or departments within a given organization or between organizations, as well as with patients and families. D'Amour and Oandasan (2005) delineated the concept of interprofessionality, part of the background work necessary for effective practice and quality outcomes, as

> the process by which professionals reflect on and develop ways of practicing that provide an integrated and cohesive answer to the needs of the client/family/population. . . . [I]t involves continuous interaction and knowledge sharing between professionals, organized to solve or explore a variety of education and care issues all while seeking to optimize the patient's participation. . . . Interprofessionality requires a paradigm shift, since interprofessional practice has unique characteristics in terms of values, codes of conduct, and ways of working. These characteristics must be elucidated. (p. 9)

Collaboration implies working together for the greater good, but it actually encompasses far more. Collaboration involves teams working on mutually developed and shared objectives. Communication must be straightforward and courteous, keeping in mind the overall intent of the objectives of the teams' work. Although collaboration has been associated with teamwork, there is more to a successful collaboration than teamwork. Effective collaboration across disciplines requires explicit, appropriate tasks and goals; clear, meaningful roles for each individual; and transparent leadership and feedback on performance (Reeves & Lewin, 2004). In an ethnographic study, Reeves and Lewin (2004) investigated interprofessional collaboration in a hospital setting. They found that the organization itself was composed of individual and isolated nursing units, and the task-oriented nature of hospital work limited opportunities for collaboration with other professionals. Consequently, collaboration tended to be task based, time limited, and formal. The lack of time, staff turnover, lack of knowledge, lack of commitment to the process, and failure to attend meetings emerged as themes in this study.

Effective interprofessional collaboration requires that team members share common perceptions and expectations of each other's roles. A systematic review of five studies on the effectiveness of interprofessional collaboration found that daily discussion, or rounds, showed a positive impact on length of stay and total financial charges and that monthly multidisciplinary team meetings improved prescription of psychotropic drugs in nursing homes (Zwarenstein, Goldman, & Reeves, 2009). Although this is beyond the scope of this chapter, an expert panel representing disciplines of nursing, medicine, pharmacy, dentistry, and public health have developed a set of core competencies for interprofessional collaborative practice. The domains include values and ethics related to interprofessional practice, roles and responsibilities of collaborative members, effective communication strategies, and the nature of teams and teamwork (https://www.aacn nursing.org/LinkClick.aspx?fileticket=8b0GriTno5Q%3d&portalid=42). See Box 1.1 for examples of interprofessional collaboration in action.

BOX 1.1

LITERATURE-BASED EXAMPLES OF INTERPROFESSIONAL COLLABORATION

Goldman, J. (2010). Interprofessional collaboration in family health teams: An Ontario-based study. *Canadian Family Physician, 56*(10), e368–e374.

McAlister, F. A., Stewart, S., Ferrua, S., & McMurray, J. J. (2004). Multidisciplinary strategies for the management of heart failure patients at high risk for admission. *Journal of the American College of Cardiology, 44*, 810–819. doi:10.1016/S0735-1097(04)01123-4

Naughton, B., Mylotte, J., Ramadan, F., Karuza, J., & Priore, R. (2001). Antibiotic use, hospital admissions, and mortality before and after implementing guidelines for nursing home-acquired pneumonia. *Journal of the American Geriatrics Society, 49*, 1020–1024. doi:10.1046/j.1532-5415.2001.49203.x

Phelan, A., Barlow, C., & Iversen, S. (2006). Occasioning learning in the workplace: The case of interprofessional peer collaboration. *Journal of Interprofessional Care, 20*(4), 415–424.

Wang, T., & Bhakta, H. (2013). A new model for interprofessional collaboration at a student-run free clinic. *Journal of Interprofessional Care, 27*(4), 339–340. doi:10.3109/13561820.2012.761598

Zwarenstein, M., & Bryant, W. (2000). Interventions to promote collaboration between nurses and doctors. *Cochrane Database of Systematic Reviews, 2000*(2), CD000072. doi:10.1002/14651858.CD000072

Reflection

Clinical wisdom implies an honesty to one's self gained through reflection on one's own practice. Reflection involves examination and an "imaginative, creative, nonlinear, human act" designed to recapture an experience and evaluate it (Ruth-Sahd, 2003, p. 488). Reflective practice allows new discoveries based in the practice situation to emerge (Durgahee, 1997). Dewey (1933) first introduced the idea of reflective practice, stating that "reflective thinking is closely related to critical thinking; it is the turning over of a subject in the mind and giving it serious and consecutive consideration" (p. 3). He noted that those who are reflective are open-minded and responsive to their experiences. According to Denner (2009), reflection causes a change in brain activity, specifically increases in alpha and theta waves. This change occurs particularly in the right hemisphere of the brain, which is associated with insight and "the sudden awareness of correct answers" (p. 326).

Professional practice is unique and complex. To practice in a professional manner requires reflection as a means of learning from experience. Schön (1983, 1990) makes a distinction among three methods of reflection: reflection-in-action, reflection-on-action, and reflection-for-action. Reflection-in-action is a spontaneous reflection in the middle of the action, essentially, "thinking on your feet" (1990, p. 26). It is a conscious, spontaneous response to a situation that may be difficult to describe when asked, but allows reflection on a situation as it is occurring. Reflection-in-action involves learning by experience and the unexpected feedback it might entail, which allows a reframing of the experience. For example, Dickson, McVittie, and Kapliashrami (2017), in a qualitative study of how community health nurses establish relationships with patients, noted that regardless of the communities within which they practiced, the participants highlighted the need for negotiation as a foundation of caring. They described taking time in establishing and maintaining trusting relationships, allowing them to elicit patient and carer expectations of the service to be provided and to identify their needs. One of the participants' descriptions related a "sense of seeking permission to care and having to negotiate 'a way in,' enabling her to work out priorities" (p. e456).

Reflection-on-action is about thoroughly reviewing a situation after it has occurred. For example, conducting a root-cause analysis following an adverse event or a debriefing with students following a simulated clinical activity represents reflection and critical thinking about actions that have already been taken. In this way, actual practice can be analyzed and alternative methods of action can be discussed, if necessary.

Reflection-for-action allows a practitioner to determine how further action will be guided. Schön believed that individual practitioners chose their own theories upon which to act, rather than blindly accepting what they were taught. He stated:

> In the varied topography of professional practice, there is a high, hard ground which overlooks a swamp. On the high ground, manageable problems lend themselves to solution through the use of research-based theory and technique. In the swampy low lands, problems are messy and confusing and incapable of technical solution. The irony of this situation is that the problems of the high ground tend to be relatively unimportant to individuals or to society at large, however great their technical interest may be, while in the swamp lie the problems of greatest human concern. (Schön, 1992, p. 54)

Ghaye and Lillyman (2014) suggest a more positive approach to reflection using *appreciative reflection*, a form of reflection that invites people to attend to the positive aspects in their relationships with others. Appreciative reflection is fueled by positive questions, such as:

- What is currently working well?
- What is right?
- What do I see as the very best in the people I work with?
- What breathes life into good working relationships?

Appreciative reflection is a practice that focuses on relating and finding the positive aspects in work situations that can be supported and nurtured through interaction (e.g., working with teams, mentoring) and dialogue. It involves caring about growth-promoting and healthcare performance-enhancing relationships. Appreciative reflection requires a commitment to building trust among interprofessional collaborative teams, being open and ready for innovation, and developing learning-enriched clinical areas.

The benefits and limitations to reflective practice include (Davies, 2012):

Benefits:
- In-depth learning from each experience or situation, including acquisition of new knowledge and skills
- Identification of personal, professional, and educational areas for improvement

- Increased understanding of one's own beliefs, attitudes, and values in varying situations
- Improvement in clinical confidence

Limitations:
- Lack of understanding of the reflective process
- Discomfort in evaluating own practice
- Time-consuming

DEVELOPING A SCHOLARLY PRACTICE

The value of understanding the complex relationships involved in nursing practice, nursing knowledge, clinical wisdom, reflection, and interprofessional practice is that knowledge grows from practice, and it is an active practice that provides the foundation for scholarly practice and, therefore, inquiry. Perhaps the single most important point in developing a scholarly practice is the desire to discover something new and then share it (Hauptman, 2005). Communities of practice, which are groups of people with a common interest and a shared passion who interact regularly, can assist in developing practice-related scholarship (Wenger, 2004). The community is built around shared knowledge, rather than a task. Active engagement by community members is essential. Learning arises out of the act of social participation and evolves through collaboration over time (Andrew, Tolson, & Fergurson, 2008). For example, a famous community of practice is the Xerox Corporation's Eureka project, which developed around customer service (Brown & Duguid, 2000). The Xerox staff began exchanging tips and tricks learned on the job at informal meetings over breakfast or lunch. Xerox saw the value of these interactions and created the Eureka project to allow these interactions to be shared across the global network of representatives. These efforts saved the corporation $100 million. In nursing, communities of practice have been used to decrease falls (Francis-Coad et al., 2018), build research capacity among advanced practice nurses (Landeen, Kirkpatrick, & Doyle, 2017), and improve smoking- cessation data collection (McCullough, Small, & Prady, 2013).

Geographic separation is not an issue, as those with shared goals in scholarship can develop or enhance a scholarly practice through the use of technology. By using technology, communities of practice can bring groups together to share expertise and enhance scholarship. For example, a community of occupational therapists met virtually to discuss cases, integrate evidence with experience, identify gaps, shape practice, and improve outcomes. Focused on community mental health, this group is composed of Canadian occupational therapists who work together to integrate a model of recovery into their practice (White, Basiletti, Carswell, & Head, 2008). The outcome of their effort was a model of best practice that is now used across Canada. Nurses, collaborating both in real time and online, formed a community of practice to address outdated practices and to promote professional development in the area of gerontology (Tolso, McAloon, Hotchkiss, & Schofield, 2005). The community developed and tested best-practice statements (www.geronurse.com).

CONCLUSIONS

Being a scholar and engaging in scholarly inquiry requires an understanding of the nature of practice, a willingness to be involved in new situations, reflection on current practice, confidence, and commitment (Riley & Beal, 2013). Developing a scholarly practice requires consideration of the following essential elements (Dyck, 2012; Lombardozzi, 2013):

■ Know what scholarly activity is about; this is an important first step. Research is only a part of scholarly activity. To begin requires reflection on the situations around us. "To put it metaphorically: A man is walking down the beach and he sees a rock. He pauses and thinks, I wonder what's under that rock?" He starts to dig and discovers a fish skeleton. The man sees another fellow walking down the beach and yells: "HEY! Want to see what's under this rock?" (Dyck, 2012, p. 1043). In other words, he makes a discovery, reflects on its importance, and seeks to disseminate his findings. Scholarly inquiry involves grounding work in theory and previous research. Scholar-practitioners must have an inquiring and analytic mind-set as they seek to learn deliberately from practice and adjust approaches to constantly improve both scholarship and practice.

■ Take an evidence-based approach to scholarly practice. Deliberately searching the literature for the evidence behind new guidelines and protocols, evaluate the strength of the evidence, and keep an eye on outcomes.

■ Be prepared to find areas for scholarship in any situation.

■ Work on something you're passionate about.

■ Turn a project into a study.

■ Find and heed a voice of wisdom—a mentor.

■ Learn the basics of Excel.

- Understand that a statistician (or librarian) is your friend.
- Remember that achieving statistical significance the first time is cause for celebration.
- Write one page (or one paragraph or one sentence) a day of the final report or manuscript will keep stress away.
- Scholarly activity begets new scholarly opportunities.

■ QUESTIONS FOR DISCUSSION

1. In what ways has practice in the profession changed over the last two decades? How is it expected to change in the future?
2. What types of practice demand more attention to scholarship?
3. How does the doctor of nursing practice (DNP) degree support or inform practice changes?
4. In your opinion, is the DNP degree the logical result of the evolution of a profession?
5. What is the difference between being a student and being a scholar?

■ REFLECTIVE EXERCISES

1. Think about a new practice situation you experienced recently. To reflect on your experience, complete these sentences:
   - "I felt . . ."
   - "I was most anxious about . . ."
   - "I expected my colleagues to . . ."
   - "I learned . . ."
   - "Next time, I will . . ."
   - "I would like to inquire about . . ."
   Review your answers to see whether any of them can be further understood by a scholarly inquiry project.
2. Spend a few minutes thinking about your last year in school. What were your goals then? What were your priorities? Have your priorities changed since then?
3. Reflect on your work situation using appreciative reflection. Ask yourself:
   - What situations have you been in in which you thought that your actions worked well?
   - What strengths do you feel you have to deal with difficult situations at work?

TABLE 1.2

Goal*	What specific aims do you want to accomplish?*	How will you accomplish each of these aims?	What resources or new knowledge will you need to accomplish the specific aims and realize the goal?	Will you need a mentor? Can you identify someone?	What will be the primary outcomes and how will they be disseminated?	How long will it take to achieve each aim and meet the goal?

*You may want to make a separate column for each aim.

4. Create a plan for the development of your scholarship over the next 5 years. What do you hope to accomplish, what are your goals, and how will you achieve these goals? Use the suggested questions as a guideline.

■ SUGGESTED READINGS

Carper, B. A. (1978). Fundamental patterns of knowing in nursing. *Advances in Nursing Science, 1*(1), 13–23. doi:10.1097/00012272-197810000-00004

Kitson, A. (2006). From scholarship to action and innovation. *Journal of Advanced Nursing, 55*(5), 543–545. doi:10.1111/j.1365-2648.2006.04004_2.x

Rolfe, G. (2005). The deconstructing angel: Nursing reflection and evidence based practice. *Nursing Inquiry, 12*(2), 78–86. doi:10.1111/j.1440-1800.2005.00257.x

■ REFERENCES

American Association of Colleges of Nursing. (2017). Defining scholarship for the discipline of nursing. Retrieved from http://www.aacnnursing.org/News-Information/Position-Statements-White-Papers/Defining-Scholarship

American Association of Critical-Care Nurses. (2016). *AACN standards for establishing and sustaining healthy work environments: A journey to excellence* (2nd ed.). Aliso Viejo, CA: Author.

Andrew, N., Tolson, D., & Ferguson, D. (2008). Nurse education today building on Wenger: Communities of practice in nursing. *Nurse Education Today, 28*(2), 246–252.

Benner, P. (1994). *Interpretive phenomenology: Embodiment, caring, and ethics in health and illness*. Thousand Oaks, CA: Sage.

Benner, P., Hooper-Kyriakidis, P., & Stannard, D. (2011). *Clinical wisdom and interventions in critical care* (2nd ed.). Philadelphia, PA: Saunders.

Bradley, E. H., Curry, L. A., & Devers, K. J. (2007). Qualitative data analysis for health services research: Developing taxonomy, themes, and theory. *Health Services Research*, 2(4), 1758–1772. doi:10.1111/j.1475-6773.2006.00684.x

Brown, J. S., & Duguid, P. (2000, May–June). Balancing act: How to capture knowledge without killing it. *Harvard Business Review*. Retrieved from https://pdfs.semanticscholar .org/efd3/009792a3f48ffe5c579306dfc07fee5b5dfa.pdf

Carper, B. A. (1978). Fundamental patterns of knowing in nursing. *Advances in Nursing Science*, 1(1), 13–23. doi:10.1097/00012272-197810000-00004

D'Amour, D., & Oandasan, I. (2005). Interprofessionality as the field of interprofessional practice and interprofessional education: An emerging concept. *Journal of Interprofessional Care*, 19(Supplement 1), 8–20. doi:10.1080/13561820500081604

Davies, S. (2012). Embracing reflective practice. *Education for Primary Care*, 23(1), 9–12. doi:10.1080/14739879.2012.11494064

Denner, S. S. (2009). The science of energy therapies and contemplative practice. A conceptual review and application of zero balancing. *Holistic Nursing Practice*, 23(6), 315–334. doi:10.1097/HNP.0b013e3181bf3784

Dewey, J. (1933). *How we think: A restatement of the relation of reflective thinking to the educative process* (2nd ed.). New York, NY:D. C. Heath.

Dickson, C. A. W., McVittie, C., & Kapilashrami, A. (2017). Expertise in action: Insights into the dynamic nature of expertise in community-based nursing. *Journal of Clinical Nursing*, 27(3–4), e451–e462. doi:10.1111/jocn.13950

Dossey, B. M., Keegan, L., & Guzzetta, C. E. (2003). *Holistic nursing: A handbook for practice*. Boston, MA: Jones & Bartlett.

Haggerty, L., & Grace, P. (2008). Clinical wisdom, the essential foundation of good nursing care. *Journal of Professional Nursing*, 24, 235–240. doi:10.1016/j.profnurs.2007.06.010

Durgahee, T. (1997). Reflective practice: Decoding ethical knowledge. *Nursing Ethics*, 4(3), 211–219. doi:10.1177/096973309700400305

Dyck, C. (2012). The scholarly path. *Canadian Family Physician*, 58(9), 1042–1043.

Francis-Coad, J., Etherton-Beer, C., Bulsara, C., Blackburn, N., Chivers, P., & Hill, A. M. (2018). Evaluating the impact of a falls prevention community of practice in a residential aged care setting: a realist approach. *BMC Health Services Research*, 18(1), 21.

Ghaye, T., & Lillyman, S. (2014). *Reflection: Principles and practices for healthcare professionals*. Bedfordshire, England: MA Healthcare Limited.

Gilgun, J. (2010). *The nature of practice in evidence-based practice*. Paper presented at the Theory Construction and Research Methodology Pre-Conference Workshop, National Council on Family Relations, Minneapolis, MN, November 3. Retrieved from http://www.scribd.com/doc/38917585/The-Nature-of-Practice-in-Evidence-Based-Practice

Girard, F., Linton, N., & Besner, J. (2005). Professional practice in nursing: A framework. *Nursing Leadership*, 18(2). Retrieved from http://www.longwoods.com/content/19028

Haggerty, L., & Grace, P. (2008). Clinical wisdom, the essential foundation of good nursing care. *Journal of Professional Nursing*, 24, 235–240. doi:10.1016/j.profnurs.2007.06.010

Hauptman, R. (2005). How to be a successful scholar: Publish efficiently. *Journal of Scholarly Publishing*, 36(2), 115–119. doi:10.3138/jsp.36.2.115

Kemmis, S. (2009). What is professional practice? Recognising and respecting diversity in understandings of practice. In C. Kanes (Eds.), *Elaborating professionalism. Innovation and change in professional education* (Vol. 5, pp. 139–165). Dordrecht, Netherlands: Springer.

Landeen, J., Kirkpatrick, H., & Doyle, W. (2017). The hope research community of practice: Building advanced practice nurses' research capacity. *Canadian Journal of Nursing Research*, 49(3), 127–136. doi:10.1177/0844562117716851

Lombardozzi, B. (2013). The SMART practice of scholarly practice. *Advances in Developing Human Resources*, 15, 296–313. doi:10.1177/1523422313487839

McAlister, F. A., Stewart, S., Ferrua, S., & McMurray, J. J. (2004). Multidisciplinary strategies for the management of heart failure patients at high risk for admission. Journal of the American College of Cardiology, 44, 810–819. doi:10.1016/S0735-1097(04)01123-4

McCullough, B., Small, N., & Prady, S. L. (2013). 1 Improving smoking cessation data collection via a health visitor community of practice. Community Practitioner, 86(5), 22–25.

McKie, A., Baguley, F., Guthrie, C., Jackson, C., Kirkpatrick, P., Laing, A., . . . Wimpenny, P. (2012). Exploring clinical wisdom in nursing education. Nursing Ethics, 19(2), 252–267. doi:10.1177/0969733011416841

Naughton, B., Mylotte, J., Ramadan, F., Karuza, J., & Priore, R. (2001). Antibiotic use, hospital admissions, and mortality before and after implementing guidelines for nursing home-acquired pneumonia. Journal of the American Geriatrics Society, 49, 1020–1024. doi:10.1046/j.1532-5415.2001.49203.x

Parse, R. (1999). Nursing: The discipline and the profession. Nursing Science Quarterly, 12(4), 275–276. doi:10.1177/08943180022107924

Pearson, A. (2011). Nursing science and practical wisdom: The pillars of nursing knowledge. International Journal of Nursing Practice, 17, 443. doi:10.1111/j.1440-172X.2011.01956.x

Phelan, A., Barlow, C., & Iversen, S. (2006). Occasioning learning in the workplace: The case of interprofessional peer collaboration. Journal of Interprofessional Care, 20(4), 415–424.

Price, A. (2004). Encouraging reflection and critical thinking in practice. Nursing Standard, 18(47), 46–52. doi:10.7748/ns2004.08.18.47.46.c3664

Reeves S., & Lewin, S. (2004). Interprofessional collaboration in the hospital: Strategies and meanings. Journal of Health Services Research & Policy, 9(4), 218–225. doi:10.1258/1355819042250140

Rew, L., & Barrow, E. (1987). Intuition: A neglected hallmark of nursing knowledge. Advances in Nursing Science, 10(1), 49–62. doi:10.1097/00012272-198710000-00010

Rew, L., & Barrow, E. (1989). Nurses' intuition. Can it coexist with the nursing process. AORN Journal, 50(2), 353–358. doi:10.1016/S0001-2092(07)65985-7

Riley, J. M., & Beal, J. A. (2013). Scholarly nursing practice from the perspectives of early-career nurses. Nursing Outlook, 61(2), e16–e24. doi:10.1016/j.outlook.2012.08.010

Ruth-Sahd, L. (2003). Reflective practice: A critical analysis of data-based studies and implications for nursing education. Journal of Nursing Education, 42(11), 488–497.

Schön, D. (1983). The reflective practitioner: How professionals think in action. London, UK: Basic Books.

Schön, D. A. (1990). Educating the reflective practitioner. San Francisco, CA: Jossey-Bass.

Schön, D. A. (1992). The crisis of professional edge and the pursuit of an epistemology. Journal of Interprofessional Care, 6, 49–63. doi:10.3109/13561829209049595

Schraeder, B., & Fischer, D. (1986). Using intuitive knowledge to make clinical decisions. Journal of Maternal-Child Nursing, 11, 161–162. doi:10.1097/00005721-198605000-00002

Seiden, H. M. (2010). The wild and the wise: Searching for clinical wisdom. Psychologist-Psychoanalyst, 2010(Summer), 19–20.

Tolson, D., McAloon, M., Hotchkiss, R., & Schofield, I. (2005). Progressing evidence-based practice: an effective nursing model? Journal of Advanced Nursing, 50(2), 124–133. doi:10.1111/j.1365-2648.2005.03371.x

Uhrenfeldt, L., & Hall, E. (2007). Clinical wisdom among proficient nurses. Nursing Ethics, 14(3), 387–398. doi:10.1177/0969733007075886

Wang, T., & Bhakta, H. (2013). A new model for interprofessional collaboration at a student-run free clinic. Journal of Interprofessional Care, 27(4), 339–340. doi:10.3109/13561820.2012.761598

Wenger, E. (2004). Communities of practice and social learning systems. In K. Starkey, S. Tempest, & A. McKinlay (Eds.), How organizations learn: Managing the search for knowledge (2nd ed., pp. 238–258). London, UK: Thomson Learning.

White, C. M., Basiletti, M. C., Carswell, A., & Head, B. J. (2008). Online communities of practice: Enhancing scholarly practice using web-based technology. *Occupational Therapy Now, 10*, 6–7.

Zander, P. (2007). Ways of knowing in nursing: The historical evolution of a concept. *Journal of Theory Construction and Testing, 11*(1), 6–11.

Zwarenstein, M., & Bryant, W. (2000). Interventions to promote collaboration between nurses and doctors. *Cochrane Database of Systematic Reviews, 2000*(2), CD000072. doi:10.1002/14651858.CD000072

Zwarenstein, M., Goldman, J., & Reeves, S. (2009). Interprofessional collaboration: Effects of practice-based interventions on professional practice and healthcare outcomes. *Cochrane Database of Systematic Reviews, 2009*(3) CD000072. doi:10.1002/14651858. CD000072.pub2

CHAPTER 2

Practice-Based Scholarly Inquiry

■ OBJECTIVES

At the end of this chapter, you will be able to:

- Explain Boyer's model of scholarship.
- Explain the components of a research proposal.
- Determine the type of scholarship best suited for a particular research question.

■ KEY CONCEPTS

- Scholarship in nursing is about those activities that advance the profession.
- All scholarly inquiry starts with a question that guides the entire project.
- Developing a plan to conduct the study is an iterative process.

INTRODUCTION

Scholarship in nursing involves activities that advance the profession through teaching, research, and practice. Scholarship in nursing can occur in both the role of practitioner or faculty member. According to Boyer (1990), scholarship is generally thought to be related to research; however, the work of a real scholar involves "stepping back . . . looking for connections, building bridges between theory and practice, and communicating one's work" (p. 16)—in other words, *reflecting*. Boyer

© Springer Publishing Company DOI: 10.1891/9780826134943.0002

Teaching	Discovery
The *aesthetic* question:	The *empirical* question:
What is valuable? What is important? How do I engage?	What needs to be known? What is true?
"Teaching begins with what the teacher knows. Teachers must be well informed. It continues by educating and enticing students through transmitting knowledge as well as transforming and extending it" *(Boyer, 1990, p. 24).*	*"We take the position that research is at the very heart of academic life, and we celebrate what we call the scholarship of discovery"* *(Boyer, 1990, p. 89).*
Integration	Application
The *reality* question:	The *practical* question:
What is best practice?	How do I improve service?
"Integration is the disciplined work that makes connections among isolated works and fields, placing facts into context, interprets, and draws new insight into research" *(Boyer, 1990, p. 19).*	*"Service activities must be tied directly to one's special field of knowledge and relate to, and flow directly out of, this professional activity. Such service is serious, demanding work, requiring the rigor—and the accountability.... In application activities, theory and practice vitally interact, and one renews the other"* *(Boyer, 1990, p. 23).*

FIGURE 2.1 Scholarship.

outlined four domains of scholarship: teaching, discovery, integration, and application (Figure 2.1). Inquiry into any one of these domains can provide support for evidence-based practices, and each has a specific delineation of what comprises scholarly inquiry. See Table 2.1 for examples in each area of scholarship.

The *scholarship of discovery* is about investigation and the "advancement of knowledge" (Boyer, 1990, p. 17). The scholarship of discovery takes the form of primary empirical research and a variety of qualitative and quantitative methodologies are used, including experimental, quasi-experimental, descriptive, and exploratory case studies and ethnography as well as theory development and philosophical inquiry. The scholar asks, "What needs to be known?" and sets about to find the answer. The scholarship of discovery is a commitment to detect new

TABLE 2.1

TYPES OF SCHOLARSHIP

Scholarship Focus	Definition	Examples
Teaching	Achieving optimal learning	Mentoring or precepting students Evaluating programs Developing instructional materials Advancing learning theory through classroom inquiry Developing and testing instructional materials Mentoring doctoral student projects Mentoring new faculty Designing and implementing a program-level assessment system Assessment of student learning needs/styles Curriculum revision based on current trends and evidence Teaching awards Development of accreditation reports
Discovery	Generating new knowledge	Publishing in peer-reviewed journals Data-based presentation Producing creative work Research grants Research awards
Integration	Synthesizing knowledge for use	Conducting systematic reviews Writing a textbook Writing book chapters
Application	Addressing problems using knowledge	Serving as a consultant Assuming leadership roles in professional organizations Advising/mentoring student leaders, fostering their professional growth Publication of case studies Quality-improvement studies Operational or program grants Peer evaluation Specialty certification

Source: Adapted from American Association of Colleges of Nursing. (1999). Defining scholarship for the discipline of nursing. *Proceedings of the AACN Task Force on Defining Standards for the Scholarship of Nursing.* Washington, DC: Author.

knowledge using well-developed and traditional methods of research. The discovery scholar asks broad questions, such as:

- What do we currently know and what do we want to know?
- What more needs to be determined? What do we want to learn more about?
- What methods and tools will work best for what we want to know and/or learn more about?

For example, Butsch-Kovacic et al. (2015) examined the pathogenesis of allergy in obese versus normal- weight children using genetic methods. They found that asthma was significantly associated with weight (odds ratio $[OR]$ = 1.38; p = 0.037). The number of genes and the magnitude of their associations with asthma were greater in overweight children alone versus normal weight and overweight children together.

The *scholarship of integration* is about synthesis, giving meaning to isolated facts, and putting them in perspective. In other words, it is about illuminating data in different ways, making connections across disciplines, and seeking to interpret findings and generate new patterns for practice. The integration of knowledge across disciplinary lines allows intercollaboration in identifying patterns, trends, and the generation of next questions that can be used by the discovery scholar. The integrative scholar asks, "What do the findings mean?" Such analysis can lead the scholar from information to knowledge and "perhaps even wisdom" (Boyer, 1990, p. 19). The broad questions necessary for integrative scholarship include:

- Can we develop an enhanced understanding of a phenomenon by synthesizing evidence across various study questions and methods?
- Can we interpret what's known to provide a more comprehensive understanding?

For example, in a systematic review of effectiveness, Holly, Porter, Kamienski, and Lim (2018) examined completed research studies on strategies used to teach gun safety to children, finding that none of the strategies were very effective.

The *scholarship of application* is about relevance and service. This element of scholarship is the most practical in that it seeks out ways in which knowledge can solve problems and serve the community, including the professional community. Application scholarship involves using available knowledge to solve practice problems or improve processes; it applies theory to practice so that practice informs theory. To be considered scholarly, service activities need to flow from professional activity, where theory and practice interact. "Practice scholarship encompasses all aspects of the delivery of nursing service where evidence of direct impact in solving healthcare problems or in defining the health problems of a community is presented. Competence in practice is the method by which knowledge in the profession is both advanced and applied" (American Association of Colleges of Nursing [AACN], 1999, para 18). The scholar asks, "How can knowledge be applied to problems, and how can I help?" Engaging in application requires using leadership skills, discipline knowledge, problem solving, and, sometimes, professional writing skills. The broad questions to be addressed by the scholarship of application include:

- How can what is known either through research or theory be applied to practice problems?
- How does the current practice problem to be addressed advance knowledge?
- What needs to be done to resolve the practice problem?

For example, Padgett, Gossett, Mayer, Chien, and Turner (2017) conducted a case study to determine how well a safety culture improved patient safety in a reliability-seeking organization. Five themes emerged from an analysis of collected data, including process standardization, checks and redundancy, authority migration, communication, and teamwork. These themes uncovered the need for extensive education and training, communication, and teamwork to improve patient safety.

The *scholarship of teaching* is the central element of all scholarship. This element recognizes the daunting work that goes into mastery of knowledge as well as the presentation of information so that others might understand it. "Teaching, at its best, means not only transmitting knowledge, but transforming and extending it as well—and by interacting with students in creative ways" (Boyer, 1990, p. 21). In this context, students also include patients. The construction of a knowledge base composed of methods, approaches, and activities designed to help assist learning, remembering, and applying subject matter is a primary focus. The identification of methods, approaches, activities, and devices faculty members use to help students understand difficult concepts for specific content or activities constitutes another important aspect of the construction of this knowledge base. The scholarship of teaching is about the study of teaching models and practices used to achieve maximum learning. Investigation into the effectiveness of untested approaches can be conducted. "The scholarship of teaching is conducted through application of knowledge of the discipline or specialty area in the teaching–learning process, the development of innovative teaching and evaluation methods, program development, learning outcome evaluation, and professional role modeling" (AACN, 1999, para 15). The scholar asks, "What works best to help my students (patients) learn?" The broad questions teaching scholars ask are:

- What teaching strategies work best under what circumstances?
- How can students best be engaged to learn?
- How can necessary knowledge be made relevant?

For example, Laurencelle, Scanlan, and Brett (2016) used qualitative methods to determine what it means to be a nurse educator. Six themes emerged:

1. Opportunities
2. Wanting to teach
3. Seeing students learn
4. Contributing to the profession
5. Difficult or negative experiences
6. Flexibility

The authors concluded that understanding how nurse educators experience academia and how the meaning of these experiences attract them to academia, facilitates the development of creative strategies to recruit and retain qualified nurse educators.

If works of scholarship in any domain are to be accepted, they need to be characterized by a clearly focused clinical question, a clear understanding of research in the field, the use of appropriate methods, and a reflective critique of the process.

A FOCUSED CLINICAL QUESTION

The decisive activity in any investigation is asking the right question, followed by writing a protocol that outlines the strategies to be used in answering the question (see Box 2.1). According to Kitchenham (2004), the right question is one that:

- Is consequential and important to both practitioners and researchers
- Will lead to changes in practice or validation of current practice
- Addresses commonly held beliefs and reality

BOX 2.1

ESSENTIAL COMPONENTS OF A PROPOSAL

Introduction
Identify the focus of the study.
Establish the significance of the study.
Discuss one or two background studies related to your topic.
State the study aims and research question.
Explain how the study is relevant to nursing practice.

Review of the Literature
Synthesize the literature on the topic.
Summarize how your study will contribute to nursing knowledge by filling in gaps and validating or testing knowledge.

Theoretical Framework
Describe the theoretical framework to be used in the study.
Connect the study aims and research questions to the theoretical framework.
Operationally define study variables.
Provide any study assumptions.

Method
Describe the study design.
Describe the setting and sample for the study, including inclusion and exclusion criteria.
Describe how the sample will be recruited, if appropriate.
Describe human subject protection methods.
Describe how data will be collected, including the validity and reliability of any instruments to be used.
Describe how data will be measured.
State anticipated findings.
State the limitations of the study.

Time Frame
Describe the time it will take to complete the study.
Provide a week-by-week listing of activities from start to completion.

Developing a research question starts with reflecting on a broad area of concern. Consider, for example, this very general question:

Is obesity a health problem in America?

This is a very broad question, known as a *foreground question*, although it provides a focus (obesity and health) and a population (Americans).

28PART I

However, it can be answered as either yes or no, which allows an opinion, but does not provide a good guide for a research study. Evidence to answer the question can be found in books, reports, or other literature and a specific investigation is not necessary. Proceeding from this point requires that the key components for the study be delineated more specifically. These key components are:

- Patient/population
- Intervention
- Comparison
- Outcome

When describing the population, it is important to describe the population of primary interest and the important characteristics of the population that are salient to the study, for example, the patient's main concern or chief complaint, health status, age, ethnicity, race, gender, and current treatment. Identifying the intervention is the second step in the patient, intervention, comparison, outcome (PICO) process. It is important to identify any treatment or intervention that will be used, for example, a new medication, a new method of brushing teeth, a new therapy, or a new procedure. The comparison is the main alternative treatment and standard of care, and it can be a different intervention, usual care, or nothing at all. The outcome is the final component of the PICO question. It describes the intended or anticipated results, and it should be measurable. Outcomes can include relief of specific symptoms, such as pain, a decrease in length of stay, or a decrease in infection. Outcomes should be as specific as possible. The PICO for the American children with obesity could be:

P = Obese Hispanic children between the ages of 13 and 17 years
I = A culturally congruent diet plan
C = Usual meal plan
O = A decease in body mass index (BMI) of 10%

The key components can now be stated as a question: In obese Hispanic children, aged 13 through 17 years, what is the effect of a culturally congruent dietary plan on basal metabolic rate (BMR)?

A PICO and its research question can also be qualitative. In this case, PICO is referred to as *PICo* for population, interest phenomenon, and context. For example, what is the meaning of retirement (I) among elderly women (P) in an adult residential community (C)? Another mnemonic that can be used for both quantitative and qualitative question development is SPICE: setting, perspective, intervention, comparison, and evaluation. For example, "In the emergency department, how do nurses interact with patients who have pain related to sickle cell disease as opposed to those with nonsickle cell pain?"

To determine whether this is a good clinical question, FINER (feasible, interesting, novel, ethical, relevant) questions can be asked. According to Hulley, Cummings, Browner, Grady, & Newman (2007), FINER questions include:

■ Feasible

Are there enough subjects? A preliminary calculation of sample size can be beneficial. There are a number of free online calculators that can help determine an adequate sample size (e.g., G-Power). If the calculated number of subjects seems too large, a number of strategies can be used to decrease this number, including expanding the inclusion criteria, lengthening the study's time frame, or recruiting another site into the study. Other important questions are:
  • Is the technical expertise available to conduct the study?
  • Is the study affordable in time and money?
  • Is the study manageable in scope?

■ Interesting

Are there others in addition to the researcher who find the question interesting? The researcher should speak with mentors, advisors, outside experts or funding agencies before developing a project around a topic that others might consider tedious or not relevant.

■ Novel

Does the study confirm, extend, or refute previous study? Does the study apply theory to practice in new ways? Are new methodological approaches being used?

■ Ethical

Is the study amenable to institutional review board guidelines? If a study has unacceptable physical or emotional risks or invades privacy, it should not be conducted. The researcher will need to seek other ways to investigate the topic.

■ Relevant

Is the study relevant to practice, policy, or further research? How will the findings of the study inform or advance practice or policy or guide research?

APPROACHES TO SCHOLARLY INQUIRY

Scholarly inquiry takes one of three approaches: quantitative, qualitative, or mixed method—a combination of the two approaches (Table 2.2). The choice of a strategy for inquiry is dependent upon the focus of the study. Is the focus an in-depth understanding (qualitative), a need to infer cause and effect (quantitative), or both (mixed method)?

Qualitative inquiry is a general term for types of research methods, such as ethnography, grounded theory, phenomenology, or participant observation research. It emphasizes the importance of the natural setting. Exhaustive data are gathered through interviews using open-ended questions that provide direct quotations. The interviewer is an integral part of the investigation and is considered the research tool. This differs from the quantitative approach, which gathers data by objective

TABLE 2.2

QUALITATIVE VERSUS QUANTITATIVE APPROACHES TO INQUIRY

Characteristic	Quantitative	Qualitative
Purpose	Prediction, control, description, confirmation, hypothesis testing Generalizability	Understanding of social phenomena through words and pictures Interpretation
Focus	Precise but narrow outcomes	Holistic process
Design	Predetermined	Emergent
Tools	Instruments (scales, tests, surveys, questionnaires, computers)	The human investigator
Data	Objective	Subjective
Conditions	Artificial	Naturalistic
Advantages	Unbiased	More in-depth description of events, feelings, perceptions, experiences
Disadvantages	Lacks in-depth information	Lacks reliability and validity Potential for researcher bias
Researcher role	Detached	Personal involvement

methods, such as surveys or physiological measurements, to provide information about effects, associations, comparisons, and predictions. In the quantitative approach, the investigator is remote from the data.

A qualitative approach is constructivist in nature (experiential thinking) and collects open-ended, emerging data with the intent of developing themes. Qualitative research uses detailed descriptions from the perspective of the research participants as a means of examining a phenomenon. The qualitative method is about exploring issues, perceptions, feelings, and experiences and understanding social phenomena. It is nonstatistical.

Qualitative inquiry is an inductive process in which themes and categories emerge from the data. Samples are usually small, often less than 10, and are often purposively selected. Purposive sampling is an essential feature of qualitative inquiry, in which subjects are selected based on some characteristics, such as gender, ethnicity, or having a certain condition, such as asthma. For example, a researcher may be interested in the at-home experiences of elderly Medicare beneficiaries with heart failure who are readmitted within 90 days of discharge from an acute care facility. The usual procedure in a qualitative study is to:

- Write the research question and select a qualitative strategy of inquiry.
- Identify the researcher role.
- Describe the selection and assignment process of participants.
- Specify methods of collecting and recording of data.
- Identify the steps in analyzing and coding the qualitative data to generate themes.

A quantitative approach is one in which the scholar takes a primarily postpositive view to develop knowledge (reductionist thinking), collect data using surveys or other instruments that yield data for statistical analysis, and analyze the collected data using statistical techniques. Quantitative inquiry is about measurement, such as attitudes, satisfaction, laboratory values, physiological parameters, or anything that can be reduced to a number. Quantitative research tests theory. For example, what are the most important factors that influence a patient's choice of a primary care provider? The usual procedure for a quantitative study is to:

- Write the research question and identify the type of design.
- Identify the population and sample.
- Describe the recruitment, selection, and assignment process of participants.

- Identify the instrument and report validity and reliability.
- Specify the major variables.
- Provide definition of terms.
- Identify how validity is addressed in the design.
- Describe the statistical tests to be used for data analysis.

A mixed-method approach combines qualitative and quantitative approaches. A rationale is developed for mixing the types of data at each stage of the inquiry (Creswell, 2003).

The decision as to which of the approaches to use is based on the type of question to be asked. It is important to clarify the type of question you are asking so that the best research design can be used. Types of questions can be categorized as "therapy" (i.e., treatment, interventions), "diagnosis" (i.e., the selection and interpretation of diagnostic tests), "etiology" (i.e., causation), "prognosis" (i.e., the effect or impact of a disease or condition), "harm" (consequences of disease or treatment), or "meaning" (Table 2.3).

REFLECTIVE CRITIQUE

To reflect critically on one's work is an essential activity in developing as a scholar, both in terms of process and outcomes. The essential question to ask is, "What would I do differently next time?" In addition, the following questions can guide a reflective critique.

- How can I use the results of this project to improve my practice?
- What will I do next in terms of researching this topic?
- What facilitated my work?
- What challenges were encountered and were they amicably resolved?

CONCLUSIONS

Scholarship is defined as the discovery, integration, application, and teaching of knowledge. To be recognized as scholarship, activities must be guided by a focused clinical question, informed by current knowledge in the field, and follow established methods. Importantly, results must be shared with others.

Engaging in scholarly inquiry to advance nursing practice involves commitment, leadership, acceptance of challenges, and integration

TABLE 2.3

SUGGESTED DESIGNS USED TO ANSWER QUESTIONS

Type of Question	Study Design
Therapy	Randomized controlled trials Nonrandomized trials Cohort study Case-control study
Diagnosis/screening	Randomized controlled trials Nonrandomized trials Cohort study Case-control study
Etiology	Controlled trials Cohort study
Prognosis	Randomized controlled trials Nonrandomized trials Cohort study Case-control study
Harm	Randomized controlled trials Nonrandomized trials Cohort study Case- control study
Meaning	Case study Ethnography Grounded theory Action research Phenomenology

of evidence into practice. This includes those activities that are "(1) significant to the profession, (2) creative, (3) can be documented, (4) can be replicated or elaborated, and (5) can be peer-reviewed through various methods" (AACN, 1999, para 5). In addition, there is a responsibility for the advanced practice nurse not only to observe, describe, understand, and assess clinical phenomena through theoretical and empirical knowledge, but also to translate best evidence and to evaluate the impact on health outcomes (Magyary, Whitney, & Brown, 2006).

■ QUESTIONS FOR DISCUSSION

1. Think about how you learn best. How would you use this knowledge to determine which domain of scholarship is best for you?
2. What criteria would you use to assess good scholarship in any of the domains?

■ REFLECTIVE EXERCISES

1. Rewrite the following questions into their PICO components. Then determine the FINER criteria for each one:
   - What is the relationship between depression and delirium?
   - Does eating fish contribute to a healthier heart?
   - Can simulated experiences increase self-confidence?
   - Does pet therapy decrease length of stay?
   - Does increased intravenous fluids work when treating patients with severe burns?
2. Think about your advanced practice situation. What areas do you think need further investigation? What theoretical framework will inform the investigation?

■ SUGGESTED READINGS

American Association of Colleges of Nursing. (1999). Defining scholarship for the discipline of nursing. *Proceedings of the AACN Task Force on Defining Standards for the Scholarship of Nursing*. Washington, DC: Author. Retrieved from http://www.aacn.nche.edu/publications/position/defining-scholarship

Morrison, C. (2012). "Boyer reconsidered": Fostering students' scholarly habits of mind and models of practice. *International Journal for the Scholarship of Teaching and Learning*, 6(1), 1–15. Retrieved from http://www.georgiasouthern.edu/ijsotl

■ REFERENCES

American Association of Colleges of Nursing. (1999). Defining scholarship for the discipline of nursing. *Proceedings of the AACN Task Force on Defining Standards for the Scholarship of Nursing*. Washington, DC: Author.

Boyer, E. L. (1990). *Scholarship reconsidered: Priorities of the professoriate*. Stanford, CA: Carnegie Foundation for the Advancement of Teaching.

Butsch-Kovacic, M., Bartin, L. J., Biagini Myers, J. M., He, H., Linsey, M., Mersha, T. B., & Khurana Hershey, G. K. (2015). Genetic approach identifies distinct asthma pathways in obese vs. normal weight children. *Allergy*, 70(8), 1028–1032. doi:10.1111/all.12656

Creswell, J. (2003). *Research design: Qualitative, quantitative and mixed method approaches*. Thousand Oaks, CA: Sage.

Holly, C., Porter, S., Kamienski, M., & Lim, A. (2018). The effectiveness of school-based and community-based gun safety educational strategies for sustained injury prevention among children aged 3-18 years: A systematic review. *Health Promotion Practice, 20*(1), 38–47.

Hulley, S. B., Cummings, S. R., Browner, W. S., Grady, D. G., & Newman, T. B. (2007). *Designing clinical research* (3rd ed.). Philadelphia, PA: Lippincott Williams & Wilkins.

Kitchenham, B. (2004). *Procedures for systematic reviews: Joint technical report*. Retrieved from http://www.inf.ufsc.br/~aldo.vw/kitchenham.pdf

Laurencelle, F., Scanlan, J., & Brett, A. L. (2016). The meaning of being a nurse educator and nurse educators' attraction to academia. *Nurse Education Today, 39*(4), 135–140. doi:10.1016/j.nedt.2016.01.029

Magyary, D., Whitney, J., & Brown, M. (2006). Advancing practice inquiry: Research foundations of the doctor of nursing practice. *Nursing Outlook, 54*(3), 139–142. doi:10.1016/j.outlook.2006.03.004

Padgett, J. D., Gossett, K., Mayer, R., Chien, W., & Turner, F. (2017). Improving patient safety through high reliability organizations. *Qualitative Report, 22*(2), 410–425.

CHAPTER 3

The DNP Project

■ OBJECTIVES

At the end of this chapter, you will be able to:

- Explain the need for the doctor of nursing practice (DNP) degree.
- Differentiate among research, quality improvement (QI), and evidence-based practice (EBP) as it relates to the practice of a nurse with a DNP degree.
- Define *practice inquiry* as it relates to the scholarship of application.
- Construct a DNP capstone proposal.
- Determine whether a project idea meets the criteria for a DNP project.

■ KEY CONCEPTS

- DNP projects reflect the mastery of the discipline acquired during doctoral education.
- The projects can take different forms, such as policy development, program evaluation, or systematic review, to identify best practice for implementation, but generally they fall under the umbrella of QI or EBP.

INTRODUCTION

DNP is a clinical practice doctorate developed to prepare practice-scholars who are "experts in specialized advanced nursing practice"

© Springer Publishing Company DOI: 10.1891/9780826134943.0003   37

(American Association of Colleges of Nursing [AACN], 2006, p. 2). The graduate of a DNP program is expected to have the necessary knowledge, skills, and attitudes to translate evidence into practice, lead QI activities, and engage in organizational and policy-change initiatives that improve patient outcomes at the local level (AACN, 2006, 2017). In other words, the DNP-prepared nurse needs to be skilled in strategies and knowledge that reduce the lag time between discovery of knowledge and its implementation in practice. The dissemination of this knowledge to larger audiences is expected.

The DNP degree is the natural evolution of a practice profession and is guided by scientific evidence, a focus on the human response, and determinants of health (Berkowitz, 2014). With the current national focus on the *Triple Aim* of reducing costs, population health, and improving patient experiences, the nurse with a DNP degree has an important role to play as part of a high-functioning healthcare team. A practice-focused doctorate ensures nursing's most skilled professionals are prepared with the similar academic rigor as other health professionals with doctoral degrees who comprise these teams, such as doctor of podiatric medicine (DPM), doctor of dental medicine and surgery (DDS), doctor of pharmacy (PharmD), doctor of physical therapy (DPT), doctor of occupational therapy (DOT), and doctor of psychology (PsyD; AACN, 2017).

The development of a practice doctorate for nurses was fueled by the increasingly complex interventions needed for patient care, national concerns about the quality of care and patient safety, shortages of doctorally prepared nursing faculty, and increasing educational expectations for the preparation of other members of the healthcare team (AACN, 2017). The DNP curriculum is grounded in AACN's DNP Essentials. These essentials outline the foundational competencies that are core to all advanced nursing practice roles, including the four nationally recognized advanced practice registered nursing roles: nurse practitioners, clinical nurse specialists, nurse anesthetists, and nurse midwives. The DNP curriculum has two components:

1. DNP Essentials one through eight provide the foundational outcome competencies deemed indispensable for all graduates of a DNP program regardless of specialty or role focus (Box 3.1).
2. Specialty content prepares the DNP graduate for practice in one of the four advanced practice roles. This specialty content is defined by the appropriate specialty organization.

BOX 3.1

DNP ESSENTIALS

Essential I: Scientific Underpinnings for Practice
A variety of sciences provide a foundation for nursing practice, including nursing science, human biology, genomics, therapeutics, psychosocial sciences, and the science of complex organizations. In addition, an understanding of philosophical, ethical, and historical issues is necessary to create a context for the application of the natural, social, and nursing sciences.

Essential II: Organizational and Systems Leadership for Quality Improvement and Systems Thinking
The DNP graduate should be prepared with expertise in assessing organizations, identifying systems' issues, and facilitating organization-wide changes in practice delivery. Advanced nursing practice requires political skills, systems thinking, and the business and financial acumen needed for the analysis of practice quality and costs.

Essential III: Clinical Scholarship and Analytical Methods for Evidence-Based Practice
The DNP graduate engages in the scholarship of application. This application involves the translation of research into practice and the dissemination and integration of new knowledge. This requires competence in the translation of research into practice, the evaluation of practice, and the use of analytic methods to critically appraise existing literature and other evidence to determine and implement the best evidence for practice. The DNP graduate should be able to design and evaluate evidence-based interventions, predict and analyze outcomes, and examine patterns of behavior and outcomes.

Essential IV: Information Systems/Technology and Patient Care Technology for the Improvement and Transformation of Healthcare
Knowledge and skills related to information systems/technology and patient care technology prepare the DNP graduate to apply new knowledge, manage individual- and aggregate-level information, and assess the efficacy of patient care technology. DNP graduates can design, select, and use information systems/technology to evaluate programs of care, outcomes of care, and care systems.

Essential V: Healthcare Policy for Advocacy in Healthcare
DNP graduates are prepared to design, influence, and implement healthcare policies that frame healthcare financing, practice regulation, access, safety, quality, and efficacy.

(continued)

BOX 3.1 (CONTINUED)

Essential VI: Interprofessional Collaboration for Improving Patient and Population Health Outcomes
DNP graduates need preparation in methods of effective team leadership and are prepared to establish interprofessional teams, participate in the work of the team, and assume leadership of the team.

Essential VII: Clinical Prevention and Population Health for Improving the Nation's Health
DNP graduates engage in leadership to integrate and institutionalize evidence-based clinical prevention and population health services for individuals, aggregates, and populations and to analyze epidemiological, biostatistical, occupational, and environmental data.

Essential VIII: Advanced Nursing Practice
A DNP graduate is prepared for advanced practice in an area of nursing specialization.

Source: American Association of Colleges of Nursing. (2006). *The essentials of doctoral education for advanced nursing practice.* Retrieved from http://www.aacnnursing.org/Portals/42/Publications/DNPEssentials.pdf

It is important to note that the DNP graduate is a scholar, one who has "gained mastery" in a specific subject area. At the end of their educational process, students complete a final scholarly project, most commonly called a *DNP capstone project*, although many other names are also used. These projects reflect the mastery of the discipline acquired during doctoral education and demonstrate the necessary engagement for practice scholarship that will influence healthcare outcomes in the practice setting. The project is in alignment with the DNP Essentials in that it is a synthesis of the student's work. The project can take different forms, such as policy development, program evaluation, or systematic review, to identify best practice for implementation, but generally they fall under the umbrella of QI or EBP.

The DNP capstone project is a form of practice inquiry. *Practice inquiry,* as defined by Magyary, Whitney, and Brown (2006), is "the ongoing, systematic investigation of questions about practice and therapeutics with the intent to evaluate and translate, as appropriate, all forms of 'best evidence' into practice and to evaluate the influence on health care outcomes" (p. 143). DNP projects include evidence appraisal and synthesis to determine what is "best evidence" that can be found in both research and clinical literature. The ability to synthesize this knowledge for practice is an essential skill for the DNP-prepared

APRN functioning in a clinical environment whose focus is on improving health and healthcare systems (M. A. Brown & Crabtree, 2013).

THE DNP CAPSTONE

The DNP capstone is not considered research; rather its focus is on EBP or QI. Research, EBP, and QI vary in structure, intent, processes, outcome, and data requirements (Table 3.1), although all are similar in that they:

- Are focused on a specific area.
- Start with a question, purpose, or concern.
- Deal with data.
- Conduct an analysis.
- Disseminate findings.

Research

Research in nursing is theory based and designed to answer a question, test an intervention, or solve a problem. The goal is to generate new knowledge. Nurse researchers follow a cycle of asking questions, setting a hypothesis, testing, and asking more questions. (See Table 3.2 for an example.) However, research is not about inquiry into practice that allows translation or application in practice situations. The Agency for Healthcare Research and Quality (2011) posits that it takes a decade or two for sustainable improvements evidenced by research findings to be used in practice.

If you can answer yes to the following questions, your project is a research study:

- Do you have a hypothesis?
- Did you search for literature that supports your hypothesis?
- Are you testing a theory or developing a new model?

Evidence-Based Practice

EBP is the integration of clinical expertise, patient values, and the best evidence into the decision-making process for patient care. The most

TABLE 3.1

EXAMPLES OF RESEARCH, EVIDENCE-BASED PRACTICE, AND QUALITY IMPROVEMENT

Focus	Description	Outcome	Example
Research	Generates new knowledge through the application of basic scientific principles and theory development. Its overall intent is to describe, predict, and control. A research study asks, "What is not known?"	Scientific knowledge that can be generalized in appropriate patient populations	Kolanowski, A. M., Hill, N. L., Kurum, E., Fick, D. M., Yevchak, A. M., Mulhall, P., . . . Valenzuela, M. (2014). Gender differences in factors associated with delirium severity in older adults with dementia. *Archives of Psychiatric Nursing, 28*(3), 187–192. doi:10.1016/j.apnu.2014.01.004
Quality improvement	Evaluates specific system's strengths and limitations, system's parts, and resulting outcomes. Asks, "What is happening?" and "How can it be improved?"	Changes that will lead to better patient outcomes and better system performance	Mileski, M., Topinka, J. B., Lee, K., Brooks, M., McNeil, C., & Jackson, J. (2017). An investigation of quality improvement initiatives in decreasing the rate of avoidable 30-day, skilled nursing facility-to-hospital readmissions: A systematic review. *Clinical Interventions in Aging, 25*(12), 213–222. doi:10.2147/CIA.S123362
Evidence-based practice	Integrates knowledge generated by research into clinical practice. An evidence-based practice project asks, "What can be done with what we know?"	Improvement in patient and system outcomes, including organizational outcomes	Brown, C. G. (2014). The Iowa model of evidence-based practice to promote quality care: An illustrated example in oncology nursing. *Clinical Journal of Oncology Nursing, 18*(2), 157–159. doi:10.1188/14.CJON.157-159

common definition of EBP was developed by Sackett, Rosenberg, Gray, Haynes, and Richardson (1996). They stated that EBP is "the conscientious, explicit and judicious use of current best evidence in making decisions about the care of the individual patient. It means integrating individual clinical expertise with the best available external clinical evidence from systematic research" (Sackett et al., 1996). Patient encounters that generate questions about the effects of therapy, the use of diagnostic tests, the prognosis, and/or the etiology of disorders provide the foundation of EBP projects.

Clinical expertise refers to the clinical provider's experience, education, and skill. Patients have personal preferences, expectations, and values that need to be incorporated into the clinician's skill set. If these preferences cannot be incorporated, a discussion needs to ensue between the provider and the patient(s) as to the reasons and alternatives need to be addressed. Best evidence for integration is determined through appraisal and synthesis of relevant, completed research studies. Evidence-based projects occur locally. They are not generalizable beyond the original setting or organization because of the contextual, unique characteristics of each setting, which cannot be controlled for in an EBP project. (See Table 3.2 for an example.)

There are several steps to the EBP process:

1. *Assess.* Clinical problems in need of resolution always start with the patient and concerns regarding experiences, the effects of therapy, the use of diagnostic tests, the prognosis and/or etiology of disorders, or the environment in which care takes place.
2. *Ask.* Construct a focused clinical question derived from the assessment using the PICO format. PICO is a mnemonic used to develop a well-focused question. The question needs to address the *p*atient, *i*ntervention, *c*omparison, and *o*utcome.

P = Patient: Describe the patient, which can include gender, age, or race of a patient if relevant to the diagnosis or treatment of a disease. For example, *families of adults in a critical care unit.*

I = Intervention: What do you want to do for the patient? Prescribe a drug? Order a test? For example, *use of bedside rounds to provide information about the patient.*

C = Comparison: What alternative treatment can the intervention be compared to? Are you trying to decide between two

TABLE 3.2

RESEARCH VERSUS EVIDENCE-BASED PRACTICE VERSUS QUALITY IMPROVEMENT

Quality Improvement	Evidence-Based Practice	Research
Identify a process or issue in need of improvement.	Identify a clinical problem in need of resolution.	Propose a hypothesis or ask a question.
Find a benchmark or collect baseline data for later comparison.	Critically appraise the literature to identify potential methods for resolution.	Design a study using the appropriate traditional research study design, such as a randomized controlled trial.
Plan an approach using one of the quality improvement models, such as PDSA .	Plan an approach using one of the evidence-based practice frameworks, such as the John Hopkins Model or the PARiHS model.	Develop a recruitment plan and select appropriate tools for data collection.
Collect the data.	Intervene and collect outcome data.	Collect the data.
Identify strategies for improvement; plan for continuing monitoring.	Develop new practice guidelines based on the evidence; plan for sustainability.	Analyze the data and interpret its meaning.
Share the findings with appropriate internal stakeholders.	Apply the evidence to practice.	Report the findings.
Act on the findings.	Evaluate the outcome.	Apply the findings to practice. PARiHS, Promoting Action on Research Implementation; PDSA, plan–do–study–act.

Source: Raines, D. A. (2012). Quality improvement, evidence-based practice, and nursing research . . . Oh my! *Neonatal Network, 31*(4), 262–264. doi:10.1891/0730-0832 .31.4.262

diagnostic tests? For example, *patient-centered conference with healthcare team versus bedside rounds*.

O = Outcome: What do you hope to accomplish? What are you trying to do for the patient? Relieve or eliminate the symptoms? Reduce the number of adverse events? For example, *achieve family satisfaction*.

PICO Question*: Among family members with an adult in the critical care unit, what is the best method of providing patient information to the family to ensure family satisfaction with care: bedside rounds versus patient care conferences?*

3. *Acquire*. A search of the literature is necessary to find answers to clinical questions. Choosing the best resource to search is an important decision. Large databases, such as Medline (Medical Literature Analysis and Retrieval System Online), will give you access to the primary literature. Secondary resources, such as Essential Evidence, will provide you with an assessment of the original study. The Cochrane and Joanna Briggs Libraries provide access to systematic reviews that have synthesized primary studies and determined a best practice.

4. *Appraise*. Appraise selected studies for validity (truth) and applicability (usefulness) using tools validated for this purpose. See, for example, the CASP (Critical Appraisal Skills Programme) tools found at https://casp-uk.net. This set of eight critical appraisal tools is designed to be used when reading research. The tools are based on the design of the research study and are used to appraise systematic reviews, randomized controlled trials, cohort studies, case-control studies, economic evaluations, diagnostic studies, qualitative studies, and clinical prediction rules. They are free to download and use under the Creative Commons License.

5. *Apply*. Integrate the best evidence found through appraisal with clinical judgment and expertise and patient preferences and implement it in practice. Decide upon an intervention or a comparison of interventions.

6. *Assess Again*. Evaluate your outcomes and determine whether your original goal or aim was met.

If you can answer yes to the following questions, your project is an EBP project:

■ Have you identified a problem in need of resolution?

■ Do you have a systems or population focus?
■ Are you considering an intervention?

Quality Improvement

QI uses a cyclical process to improve processes and find solutions for clinical problems. The Health Resources and Services Administration (2011) defines *QI* as "continuous actions that lead to measurable improvement in healthcare services and the health status of targeted patient groups" (p. 1). (See Table 3.2 for an example.) If you are able to answer yes to all of the following questions, your project is a QI project:

■ Are patients involved only through the use of a medical record review?
■ Are data being reviewed to correct deficiencies or improve a process?
■ Is there a continuous monitoring process?
■ Are a set of standards, benchmarks, or guidelines used for comparison?
■ Is immediate feedback provided to stakeholders during and after the project?

Boyer's criteria can be used to determine whether any project falls within the area of scholarship (Box 3.2).

BOX 3.2

BOYER'S CRITERIA FOR EVALUATION OF SCHOLARSHIP IN ANY DOMAIN

1. Are the aims, objectives, or goals of the project clearly stated?
2. Are the methods and procedures clearly defined and appropriate for the project?
3. Are the resources necessary for the project adequate and feasible?
4. Is there evidence that those necessary for completion of the project have been communicated with effectively?
5. Are the results of the project clinically or statistically significant?
6. Is there evidence of self-reflection and learning?

Source: Boyer, E. (1996). Clinical practice as scholarship. *Holistic Nursing Practice, 10*(3), 1–6. doi:10.1097/00004650-199604000-00003

THE DNP PROJECT

The DNP project is a culmination of the DNP program. The project is meant to reflect the knowledge and skills acquired throughout the program. A DNP project is not intended to test new models, develop new theory, or test hypotheses; rather the focus of the project is in a specific practice area of choice and is concerned with practice and/or systems issues that need resolution or greater understanding. It involves a comprehensive development plan. DNP projects:

- Focus on a change that impacts healthcare outcomes through either direct or indirect care.
- Have a systems or population focus.
- Demonstrate implementation in the appropriate arena or area of practice.
- Include a plan for sustainability (e.g., financial, systems, or political realities).
- Include an evaluation plan. DNP projects should be designed so that processes and/or outcomes will be evaluated to guide practice and policy. Clinical significance is as important in guiding practice as statistical significance is in evaluating research (AACN, 2015).

PROJECT PROPOSAL

Writing the Proposal

The purpose of writing a proposal for a research study is to provide a blueprint or plan of action that is predetermined. In this way, once the study is underway, the researcher need only to look at the proposal and follow the procedures as described. The ideas presented in the proposal must flow logically and build upon one another; in other words, the researcher builds a case for the study (Gray, Grove, & Sutherland, 2009). An outline of essential components of a research proposal is presented in Chapter 2. Every proposal should contain the following.

An *introduction* provides an opening in which to demonstrate why this is an important area of inquiry. The purpose of the study is stated and information on the background of the clinical problem and its significance are presented. Some statistics can be used to demonstrate the importance of the topic. This section should also contain the research question, the aims of the study, and a statement as to why it is necessary to investigate this issue.

A *problem statement* clearly describes the problem to be resolved. A problem statement should identify the issues and problems in the current situation, describe the context of the problems, define the magnitude of the problems using statistics and other epidemiological data as appropriate, describe the impact of the problems on the population, and provide solutions. A well-constructed problem statement provides focus for the team. The five Ws—who, what, where, when, and why—are a good tool to use to focus on the problem statement. Consider Rudyard Kipling's poem "The Elephant's Child" :

I keep six honest serving-men
(They taught me all I knew);
Their names are What and Why and When
And How and Where and Who.

Who—Who gets affected by the problem? Specific groups, organizations, stakeholders, and so on?

What—What are the boundaries or context of the problem, for example, do they involve the organization, workflow, geography, customers, segments, and so on? What impact does the problem have? What would happen when it is fixed? What would happen if it is not fixed?

When—When does the issue occur?

Where—Where is the issue occurring? Only in certain locations, processes, products, and so on?

Why—Why is it important that we fix the problem? (Lindstrom, 2009)

A *needs assessment* should be done to show support for the proposed improvement. The improvement should benefit a healthcare delivery system or population. This should include a global or national perspective as appropriate, narrowed to the project site. Publicly available data for the organization, if available, should be used. The needs assessment should detail the following:

- The population
- Stakeholders
- The organization, facility, or unit where the project will be conducted
- Available resources
- Anticipated outcomes
- Members of the team and the role of each team member
- The role of the team leader
- Scope and limitations of the project

The needs assessment should end with a statement of an overall aim or purpose of the project with specific goals that support the aim.

A *review of the literature* is the next step in writing a proposal. First, the method used to search the literature should be described, including databases searched and time frames and key words used. Salient articles should be located, critically analyzed, and synthesized. This section should describe the current state of knowledge, trends, or patterns about the topic. An explanation of how the proposed project or study will expand or validate knowledge should be included. This section does not need an annotated bibliography, but rather a thoughtful synthesis of current and relevant literature on the topic. In general, a 5-year span from the present should be used except for the inclusion of landmark or classic literature. Tables of evidence can be created from the literature review if required.

A *framework* provides an opportunity to connect the study aims and project question to a scaffold. A theory is a body of knowledge that organizes, describes, predicts, and/or explains phenomena (Sidani & Fleury, 2016). A theory that guides advanced practice should be testable and include an "integrated set of concepts, statements, relational statements, and the expected changes in outcomes" (Sidani & Fleury, 2016, p. 12). Variables should be operationally defined within the context of the theory being used, and any study assumptions should be provided. It may be useful to draw a diagram or visual map depicting the relationships among the theory's concepts and propositions and study variables and how the theory connects to the DNP project.

A *method* section that outlines methods and procedures of the study is important and should be as clear and transparent as possible. Precise detail in explaining how the data necessary to answer the project question is necessary. The study design and a justification for its use should be included. The setting, sample (including inclusion and exclusion criteria), recruitment strategies, and how human subjects will be protected need description. The method of data analysis should be explained as well as a rationale as to why the specific methods of analysis were chosen. It may be helpful to include a description of the intended outcomes and a timeline for completion so that the project stays on target.

The DNP project proposal should focus on the major elements of the plan. It should be considered a blueprint for action. The proposal should include a description of the primary goal, specific aims, rationale, expected implementation plans, and anticipated outcomes. The proposal is written in future tense using a formal writing style, such as that suggested by the American Psychological Association (APA; to review APA format, see https://owl.english.purdue.edu/owl/resource/560/01). The proposal should be about 10 to 12 pages long, exclusive of references and any appendices. It should include page numbers and a running head containing the student's last name and a very short title. A suggested outline for a capstone project is as follows:

- Cover page with the title of the project, student's name, date, and names of capstone mentors/committee
- An abstract of about 150 words; when the final project is written, this will increase to 250 to 300 words to include results and conclusions
- An introduction that introduces the problem and summarizes its significance; some background should be provided to provide substance, such as epidemiological data, cost data, or negative health outcomes data
- Focused evidence appraisal of the most relevant and current scientific work that relates to the purpose of the project; if possible, provide examples of current evidence from the literature on interventions and include an evidence table if appropriate
- Purpose and goal of the project, including PICO
- Plan for implementation that is based on the focused literature review; describe how the project will be implemented and who will be involved in the implementation
- Timeline: This should be a month-by-month description; use of a Gantt chart here is helpful
- Describe the proposed sources of information and the kind of information that will be collected in order to carry out the project
- The protection of human participants should be included, if relevant; generally, QI projects do not require application for traditional human participation; however, some kind of special form may be needed to comply with the concerned university's human participants' approval process
- Anticipated project outcome
- Potential avenues for dissemination
- References
- Appendices: Include letter of support from agency, informed consent if necessary, recruitment fliers if used, and data-collection sheets

CONCLUSIONS

To be sure that your idea for a final, culminating project meets the criteria for a DNP project, ask yourself the following questions:

- Is the focus of my project on individuals, communities, populations, and/or systems?
- Is there a specific problem or issue to be resolved?
- Will my project inform my practice or resolve a clinical issue?
- Will I be able to demonstrate mastery of DNP competencies achieved through my doctoral education?
- Is my project grounded in evidence?
- Are the outcomes of my project patient centered? (https:// www. doctorofnursingpracticednp.org/capstone-project-guide)

■ QUESTIONS FOR DISCUSSION

1. Does translating evidence into practice require a different set of skills than those used in a PhD program? In your opinion, are you learning the right set of skills to be able to change practice?
2. What challenges do you think you would face while engaging in EBP and/or QI projects in your current work setting?

■ REFLECTIVE EXERCISES

1. What is your assessment of the value of the DNP project and the role it plays in moving the profession forward? List the ways you think the project requirement can be improved. How will you share your thoughts for project improvement?
2. Think about reflection-in-action, reflection-on-action, and reflection-for-action. How can any of these concepts be used to develop a DNP capstone project?

■ SUGGESTED READINGS

Brown, M. A., & Kaplan, L. (2016). Opening doors: The practice degree that changes practice. *Nurse Practitioner, 141*(4), 35–42. doi:10.1097/01.NPR.0000481511.09489.96

Holly, C., Percy, M., Caldwell, B., Echevarria, M., Bugle, M. J., & Salmond, S. (2014). Moving evidence to practice: Reflections on a multi-site academic partnership. *International Journal of Evidence Based Healthcare, 12*(1), 31–38. doi:10.1097/XEB.0000000000000001

Moran, K. J., Burson, R., & Conrad, D. (2017). *The doctor of nursing practice scholarly project: A framework for success* (2nd ed.). Burlington, MA: Jones & Bartlett Learning.

Newland, J. (2013). DNP scholarly projects change practice. *Nurse Practitioner, 38*(4), 6. doi:10.1097/01.NPR.0000427597.86572.0d

■ REFERENCES

Agency for Healthcare Research and Quality. (2011). Fact sheet: Translating research into practice (TRIP)—II. Retrieved from https://archive.ahrq.gov/research/findings/factsheets /translating/tripfac/trip2fac.pdf

American Association of Colleges of Nursing. (2006). *The essentials of doctoral education for advanced practice nursing*. Retrieved from http://www.aacn.nche.edu/dnp/Essentials.pdf

American Association of Colleges of Nursing. (2015) *The DNP current issues and clarification recommendations*. Retrieved from https://www.pncb.org/sites/default/files/2017-02/ AACN_DNP_Recommendations.pdf

American Association of Colleges of Nursing. (2017). *The doctor of nursing practice fact sheet*. Retrieved from http://www.aacnnursing.org/Portals/42/News/Factsheets/DNP-Factsheet-2017.pdf

Berkowitz, B. (2014). The emergence and impact of the DNP degree on clinical practice. In B. A. Anderson, J. M. Knestrick, & R. Barroso (Eds.), *DNP capstone projects: Exemplars of excellence in practice* (pp. 115–127). New York, NY: Springer Publishing.

Boyer, E. (1996). Clinical practice as scholarship. *Holistic Nursing Practice, 10*(3), 1–6. doi:10.1097/00004650-199604000-00003

Brown, C. G. (2014). The Iowa model of evidence-based practice to promote quality care: An illustrated example in oncology nursing. *Clinical Journal of Oncology Nursing, 18*(2), 157–159. doi:10.1188/14.CJON.157-159

Brown, M. A., & Crabtree, K. (2013). The development of practice scholarship in DNP programs: A paradigm shift. *Journal of Professional Nursing, 29*(6), 330–337. doi:10.1016/j. profnurs.2013.08.003

Gray, J. R., Grove, S. K., & Sutherland, S. (2017). *Burns and Grove's the practice of nursing research* (8th ed.). St. Louis, MO: Elsevier.

Health Resources and Services Administration. (2011). *Quality improvement*. Retrieved from http://www.hrsa.gov/quality/toolbox/methodology/qualityimprovement

Kolanowski, A. M., Hill, N. L., Kurum, E., Fick, D. M., Yevchak, A. M., Mulhall, P., . . . Valenzuela, M. (2014). Gender differences in factors associated with delirium severity in older adults with dementia. *Archives of Psychiatric Nursing, 28*(3), 187–192. doi:10.1016/j.apnu.2014.01.004

Lindstrom, C. (2009). How to write a problem statement [Blog post]. Retrieved from www .ceptara.com/blog/how-to-write-problem-statement

Magyary, D., Whitney, J., & Brown, M. A. (2006). Advancing practice inquiry: Research foundations doctor of nursing practice. *Nursing Outlook, 54,* 139–142. doi:10.1016/j. outlook.2006.03.004

Mileski, M., Topinka, J. B., Lee, K., Brooks, M., McNeil, C., & Jackson, J. (2017). An investigation of quality improvement initiatives in decreasing the rate of avoidable 30-day, skilled nursing facility-to-hospital readmissions: A systematic review. *Clinical Interventions in Aging, 25*(12), 213–222. doi:10.2147/CIA.S123362

Sackett, D. L., Rosenberg, W. M., Gray, J. A., Haynes, R. B., & Richardson, W. S. (1996) Evidence based medicine: What it is and what it isn't. *BMJ, 312*(7023), 71–72. doi:10.1136/ bmj.312.7023.71

Sidani, S., & Fleury, J. (2016). Theory-based nursing interventions. In Henly, S. J. (Ed.), *Routledge international handbook of advanced quantitative methods in nursing research* (pp. 189–198). New York, NY: Taylor and Francis Inc.

CHAPTER 4

Finding and Appraising Best Evidence

▪ OBJECTIVES

At the end of this chapter, you will be able to:

- Search the literature to find best evidence to support a doctor of nursing practice (DNP) project.
- Articulate the steps in a critical appraisal.
- Select the appropriate critical appraisal tool based on the design of the study.
- Critically appraise a primary study or a systematic review.

▪ KEY CONCEPTS

- The quality of a DNP project is in part dependent on the credibility of the evidence that supports the project.
- A research librarian can be very helpful in refining a project search.
- A best practice for conducting literature searches is to search one electronic resource at a time. After searching the literature, the project question and inclusion and exclusion criteria may need revision.
- Critical appraisal is about establishing the quality and validity of studies for inclusion in a systematic review.
- Critical appraisal is an assessment of the benefits and strengths of research along with its flaws and weaknesses.
- Several critical appraisal tools are available for assessing the quality of evidence used to support a DNP project.

INTRODUCTION

Searching the literature for evidence to support a project and critically appraising that literature are important steps in a successful DNP project. A literature search is a comprehensive survey of publications and information on a specific topic, which results in a list of references that are used to write a literature review for the project. Conducting a literature search familiarizes you with the body of work related to the project topic. Most library websites include lists of databases and online resources (see, e.g., Dartmouth's Biomedical Libraries' Resources and Databases at www.dartmouth.edu/~library/biomed/resources/resources-full-list.html; Rutgers University libraries' indexes and databases at www.libraries.rutgers.edu/indexes). Some of these library websites offer subject guides, research guides, and toolkits/tool boxes to assist in quickly locating evidence-based information to support the DNP project question.

Critical appraisal is a careful examination of evidence to assess its reliability (dependability), worth (value), and importance (importance) in a specific context. It also provides an assessment of the benefits and strengths of research against its flaws and weaknesses.

SEARCHING THE LITERATURE

A literature search is the collecting of the research done on a topic. It provides a background for the project question. Reviewing the literature lets you see what came before and what did and did not work for others who have worked on the same topic. A literature search is done for any of the following reasons:

- To identify data sources that others have used
- To study how key concepts were measured
- To put the project in context
- To assemble evidence to support your project and findings

A literature search will be more successful with a detailed plan. First, identify key words for searching. Read several articles on the topic and note the key words and phrases used in the articles. Often a topic will have several key concepts. Generate a list of synonyms and other words that might be used to describe each concept (a concept map). These can be used as your key words for searching. A good source for choosing synonyms and search terms is the *Canadian Literacy Thesaurus* (thesaurusalpha.org/thesaurus/index.htm). It is a list of the standard terms used by cataloguers and indexers to describe literacy resources.

Next, determine what type of literature you need: primary, secondary, or tertiary. Primary literature is an original work or firsthand account describing a phenomenon or an intervention or reports of survey research. Primary literature generally includes journal articles written and reviewed by experts that are published and indexed by commercial publishers. It can also consist of prepublication prints of articles and conference proceedings or symposia. Primary literature is not filtered through interpretation or evaluation as is a systematic review. For qualitative studies, primary literature can include:

■ Letters or diaries
■ Photographs or video recordings
■ Records of organizations or government agencies (e.g., annual report, treaty, constitution, government document)
■ Speeches
■ Works of art (e.g., paintings, musical scores, buildings, poems)

Examples of primary literature include quantitative articles on target temperature management (TTM) or therapeutic hypothermia in patients after acute brain injuries (Quintard & Cariou, 2018) or cardiac arrest (Leary et al., 2013) or qualitative articles on the experience of having delirium following an orthopedic procedure (Pollard, Fitzgerald, & Ford, 2015).

Secondary literature summarizes and synthesizes primary literature. It involves the summary and/or synthesis of existing research. Secondary research is contrasted with primary research in that primary research involves the generation of data, whereas secondary research uses primary research sources as a source of data for analysis. Secondary literature, such as meta-analyses or metasyntheses, gathers all information for analysis to promote understanding or illumination of outcomes, either positive or negative, from single studies. Metastudy researchers may apply statistical methods, identifying the strength and direction of findings. For example, Sibanda, Carnes, Visentin, and Cleary (2018) synthesized the findings of 10 randomized controlled trials, reporting that music has the potential to improve outcomes of anxiety, pain, and postoperative delirium for patients undergoing hip or knee surgery.

Other sources of secondary literature include:

- Bibliographies (also considered tertiary literature)
- Commentaries or criticisms
- Magazine and newspaper articles
- Monographs

Tertiary literature highlights and/or synthesizes primary and secondary literature, allowing for summaries that might not be evident in published literature. Examples of tertiary literature are summaries on type 2 diabetes from online databases such as WebMD and DynaMed on EBSCOhost (DynaMed, 2015; Khardori, 2015). Textbooks are another example of tertiary sources because they are often based on summaries of primary or secondary literature. Other examples of tertiary literature are:

- Almanacs
- Chronologies
- Dictionaries and encyclopedias
- Directories
- Fact books
- Guidebooks
- Manuals

A best practice for conducting literature searches is to search one electronic resource at a time. Because each database will have specific features that will not be the same as those offered in other databases, relevant articles may be missed if a cross-database search is conducted. An example of a cross-database or federated search includes using Ovid to search Medline (Medical Literature Analysis and Retrieval System Online) and using Books@Ovid and the PsycINFO databases in tandem. Another example would be searching TRIP (Turning Research Into Practice; www.tripdatabase.com) or the SUMSearch (sumsearch.org) database, as both products retrieve results from a variety of sources/formats (e.g., blogs). See Box 4.1 for tips for a successful search.

CRITICAL APPRAISAL

Critical appraisal addresses broad questions related to the validity of the study results and the importance of the results to a specific population. Validity is determined by an assessment of how close the study

BOX 4.1

TIPS FOR SEARCHING DATABASES

1. Write down your project question. Base the search on one main question. Be as specific as possible.
2. Use a highlighter or make key concepts or important words in the text bold for easier recognition for use in the search statements.
3. List synonyms for the highlighted words, as some database searches may prove more effective at retrieving a larger, more relevant pool of articles if synonyms for important terms are also searched.
4. Work with a research librarian to conduct an advanced search, as an advanced search in one database may not be equivalent to an advanced search in another database. Advanced searching is a challenge that can be rewarding because it offers more control in manipulating search steps and may yield more, as well as more relevant, citation.
5. Write down all inclusion and exclusion criteria for the project. Some of the key terms can be used to focus or narrow search results.

Source: Adapted from Holly, C., Salmond, S., & Saimbert, M. (2016). *Comprehensive systematic review for advanced nursing practice.* New York, NY: Springer Publishing.

results are to reality. In studies in which the aim is to determine cause and effect, the focus of validity appraisal is on internal validity. Internal validity critical appraisal questions focus on the assignment of participants to treatments, whether participants who entered the study are sufficiently accounted for at its conclusion, whether the groups were similar at the start of the trial, whether blinding was used, and whether groups were treated ethically.

Appraisal that focuses on quantitative results ensures there is adequate reporting of data-collection methods, that analysis was appropriate, indicates whether key findings are reported appropriately, and that there is sufficient reporting of the significance and precision of the results. In quantitative research the focus is on whether all important outcomes were reported and that the benefits of the intervention versus the harms and the costs were considered. Validity of quantitative research is appraised for credibility of the researcher and credibility of methods used. In qualitative research this focus is on confirmability and dependability. Applicability questions examine whether the results can be applied to one's own practice and population of interest. In qualitative research, the aim is not to generalize but to transfer findings to situations that are contextually similar. Questions focus on the contextual similarity of results.

A major focus for appraisal of both qualitative and quantitative studies is the identification of any bias. Bias addresses the issue of believability of the findings. It is possible to have a study carried out with the highest possible standards yet still have an important risk of bias. For example, if the participant is not blinded to his or her group allocation, the study may be carried out with high quality, yet performance bias may still be an issue (Higgins & Green, 2008). See Table 4.1 for information on appraising bias.

Tools for Critical Appraisal

There are many different tools available to assess the quality of research studies within the context of a systematic review. Tools vary based on the type of design used. Checklists are most commonly used. Some other more commonly used tools are:

- CASP (Critical Appraisal Skills Programme), which provides six different critiquing tools, each based on a different type of study. These include randomized controlled trials, diagnostic, case control, cohort, economic , and qualitative studies. These are free to download and use (https://casp-uk.net/).
- CEBM (Centre for Evidence-Based Medicine) has tools available to critique diagnostic and prognostic studies and randomized controlled trials. These have been translated into Spanish, German, and Lithuanian. The tools can be accessed (www.cebm.net/critical-appraisal).
- The Jadad scoring system is a short three-question critical appraisal tool. It is used primarily for randomized controlled trials. The three questions it asks are:
  - Was the study described as randomized?
  - Was the study described as double blind?
  - Was there a description of withdrawals and dropouts?
    This scoring system can be found in the article, "Assessing the Quality of Reports of Randomized Clinical Trials: Is Blinding Necessary?" (Jadad et al., 1996).
- The Joanna Briggs Institute has a variety of critical appraisal checklists to use for qualitative studies of interpretive and critical research and for narrative, opinion, and textual papers. There are also critical appraisal tools specifically designed for randomized

TABLE 4.1

APPRAISING FOR BIAS

Type of Bias	Explanation of Bias	Critical Appraisal for Bias
Selection bias	• This results from errors in the way that research participants were selected into the study from the target population or as a result of factors that influence whether research participants remained in a study. • The intervention group is therefore different from the control/comparison group in measured or unmeasured baseline characteristics and this difference may impact prognosis or outcomes. • Also used to mean that the participants are not representative of the population of all possible participants. • There is a greater chance for selection bias with nonrandom samples or when the individual assigning participants to intervention groups has the ability to select which group the individual will be assigned to.	Randomization and allocation concealment are key to minimizing selection bias. Evaluate whether: • Randomization was used. • The allocation sequence was appropriate (such as using a random component in the sequence generation such as a random number table, coin toss, or throwing dice). • Allocation was adequately concealed.
Performance bias	• Systematic differences in care were provided to the participants in the intervention and control/comparison group. • Because of the presence of differences in the care provided, one is unable to confidently conclude that the intervention under investigation caused the effect. • Performance bias is more likely to occur if the caregiver is aware of whether a patient is in a control or treatment group. • Blinding is an approach used to prevent the subject and/or researcher/clinician from knowing the allocated intervention.	Was there blinding of subject? Was there blinding of researcher/clinician?

(continued)

TABLE 4.1 (CONTINUED)

APPRAISING FOR BIAS

Type of Bias	Explanation of Bias	Critical Appraisal for Bias
Attrition bias	• Refers to differences between control and treatment groups in terms of patients dropping out of a study or not being followed up as thoroughly as others in the various groups. • Attrition of participants from a study can produce bias if the incidence rates of people who drop out differ from those in people who complete the study. • Although dropouts will occur, readers want to be assured that missing outcome data are balanced in numbers across groups with similar reasons for missing data across groups.	Was loss due to followup (i.e., dropout, nonresponse, withdrawal, protocol deviators) reported? Did researchers apply the concept of intention to treat?
Detection (assessor or ascertainment) bias	• Occurs if outcomes are measured differently for patients depending on whether they are in the control or treatment group. • A detection bias generally occurs when the assessor (the one determining the outcome results) knows whether the subject is in the control or intervention group.	Was blinding of the assessor carried out?
Reporting bias	• Occurs when outcomes are selectively reported in the findings. • Reporting bias may occur when the assessor does not fully report all positive or negative outcomes.	How were selective outcomes reported and what was found?
Other	• Potential bias not uncovered in other domains.	Are there any other concerns identified that might indicate bias?

Source: Holly, C., Salmond, S., & Saimbert, M. (2016). *Comprehensive systematic review for advanced nursing practice.* New York, NY: Springer Publishing.

controlled trials/experimental intervention studies, cohort and case-control studies, observational studies, diagnostic studies, economic studies, and prevalence and incidence studies. (Go to http://joannabriggs.org to access the checklists.)

CONCLUSIONS

Searching the literature for relevant articles that support a DNP project is an essential step for the project's success. Articles found during the search should be critically appraised. Critical appraisal requires an understanding of the strengths and weaknesses of study design and how these impact the validity and applicability of research findings.

■ QUESTION FOR DISCUSSION

Go to the CASP website (https://casp-uk.net/). Review the critical appraisal tools found on the website. Decide which tool you would use if you were appraising a project on (a) nonpharmacological interventions to decrease delirium in postoperative care units, (b) strategies to retain nurses, (c) perceptions of patients regarding the effectiveness of over-the-counter pain medication, (d) experiences of families with a family member in critical care, (e) the characteristics and risk factors of acute delirium in hospitalized children. Choose one to appraise.

■ REFLECTIVE EXERCISE

1. Select a journal article about a research study that was analyzed using statistical techniques. Appraise the article using CATmaker. CATmaker is a software program downloadable from www.cebm.net/index.aspx?o=1216, designed to help you appraise a paper and to manipulate the outcome statistics into a useful and standard format.

■ SUGGESTED READINGS

Boccia, S., La Torre, G., Persiani, R., D'Ugo, D., van Duijn, C. M., & Ricciardi, G. (2007). A critical appraisal of epidemiological studies comes from basic knowledge: A reader's guide to assess potential for biases. *World Journal of Emergency Surgery, 2*, 7. doi:10.1186/1749-7922-2-7

Buccheri, R., & Sharifi, C. (2017). Critical appraisal tools and reporting guidelines for evidence-based practice. *Worldviews on Evidence-Based Nursing, 14*(6), 463–472. doi:10.1111/wvn.12258

Google. (2015). *Google search help. How to search on Google.* Retrieved from https://support.google.com/websearch/answer/134479?hl=en&ref_topic=3081620&vid=0-635802591522179323-4179845653

Language Center, Asian Institute of Technology. (2005, February 17). *Writing a literature review.* Retrieved from http://bertini.eng.usf.edu/pdf/literature_review.pdf

OWL at Purdue University. (2003). Sample APA papers: Literature review. Retrieved from https://library.ithaca.edu/sp/assets/users/_lchabot/sample_apa_style_litreview.pdf

■ REFERENCES

DynaMed. (2015). http://www.dynamed.com/home/

Higgins, J. P. T., & Green, S. (2008). *Cochrane handbook for systematic reviews of interventions.* West Sussex, England: Wiley-Blackwell.

Holly, C., Salmond, S., & Saimbert, M. (2016). *Comprehensive systematic review for advanced nursing practice.* New York, NY: Springer Publishing.

Jadad, A. R., Moore, R. A., Carroll, D., Jenkinson, C., Reynolds, D. J. M., Gavaghan, D. J., & McQuay, H. J. (1996). Assessing the quality of reports of randomized clinical trials: Is blinding necessary? *Controlled Clinical Trials, 17*(1), 1–12.

Khardori, R. (2018). *Type 2 diabetes mellitus.* Retrieved from https://emedicine.medscape.com/article/117853-overview

Leary, M., Grossestreuer, A. V., Iannacone, S., Gonzalez, M., Shofer, F. S., Povey, C., . . . Abella, B. S. (2013). Pyrexia and neurologic outcomes after therapeutic hypothermia for cardiac arrest. *Resuscitation, 84*, 1056–1061.

Pollard, C., Fitzgerald, M., & Ford, K. (2015). Delirium: The lived experience of older people who are delirious post-orthopaedic surgery. *International Journal of Mental Health Nursing, 24*(3), 213–221. doi:10.1111/inm.12132

Quintard, H., & Cariou, A. (2018). Targeted temperature management in severe brain-injured patient. In Ichai, C., Quintard, H., & Orban, J. C. (Eds.), *Metabolic disorders and critically ill patients* (pp. 469–477). Cham, Switzerland: Springer.

Sibanda, A., Carnes, D., Visentin, D., & Cleary, M. (2018). A systematic review of the use of music interventions to improve outcomes for patients undergoing hip or knee surgery. *Journal of Advanced Nursing.* Epub ahead of print September 19. doi:10.1111/jan.13860.

Part II

CHAPTER 5

Action Research

OBJECTIVES

At the end of this chapter, you will be able to:

- Define *action research*.
- Explain the process of action research.
- Compare action research and participatory action research (PAR).
- Select a clinical problem suitable for action research.
- Define the role of the action research facilitator.

KEY CONCEPTS

- Action research directly impacts practice.
- An aim of action research is to build capacity.
- Action research involves actively participating in a change situation.
- Action research is a cycle of data collection, reflection, and problem redefinition that is based on obtaining solutions to an identified problem.
- Action research uses a variety of qualitative and quantitative methods to collect data, although words are more important than numbers.
- Action research is a community of practice.
- The representative nature of action research grounds it in real-world practice.
- PAR is research and action done with people in communities and not done to or for them.
- PAR shifts the emphasis from action and change to collaborative research activities.

INTRODUCTION

Action research is a reflective process involving research in action. It is grounded in context and involves real-world situations and problems. It is a constantly evolving method of inquiry conducted within familiar settings by teams working together for the resolution of practice problems. The personal familiarity of the researchers with the research setting confers relevance and credibility to both the inquiry process and its findings. In other words, it is done by and with insiders—those central to and conversant with the areas to be researched (Herr & Anderson, 2005). Rather than dwelling on the theoretical, action research allows practitioners to address those real-life concerns over which they can exhibit some influence and have the ability and authority to make needed change (Ferrance, 2000). However, some amount of knowledge is always gained through action, which implies that action research is also empirical in its processes, yet different. Experimental research, for example, is about manipulation and control using causal models. In action research, when interventions are initiated the same level of control is not possible. The researcher uses observation and interviews as key data-collection approaches (Kock, 2011). For example, Aylward, Murphy, Colmer, and O'Neill (2010) observed and interviewed parents over an 18-month period to determine the success of an intervention targeted toward parents of children with attachment issues aged birth to 5 years .

Reason and Bradbury (2007) refer to *action research* as a "democratic process concerned with developing practical knowledge" (p. 1). Action research is known by a variety of other names as well (Box 5.1), although for the purposes of this chapter, the term *action research* will be used. In essence, action research is a deliberate, solution-oriented investigation characterized by a circular process of problem identification, data collection, analysis, reflection, data-derived action, evaluation, further reflection, and problem redefinition (Kemmis & McTaggart, 1988). The underlying principle is one of change and redirection as determined by continual reflection on data gathered and actions taken and by proceeding through the cycle as many times as necessary to find a solution (Figure 5.1). It is not the linear approach attributed to the scientific method. In this sense, action research resembles the nursing process and its steps of assessing, planning, implementing, evaluating, and replanning (Glasson, Change & Bidwell, 2008).

To illustrate, suppose that an investigation was conducted within an acute care hospital to examine the increasing number of patients being held in the emergency department (ED) who were awaiting

BOX 5.1

SYNONYMS FOR *ACTION RESEARCH*

Action science
Appreciative inquiry
Collaborative research
Community-based action research
Community-engaged research
Community-of-practice research
Cooperative inquiry
Developmental action inquiry
Participatory action research
Practitioner research
Praxis intervention

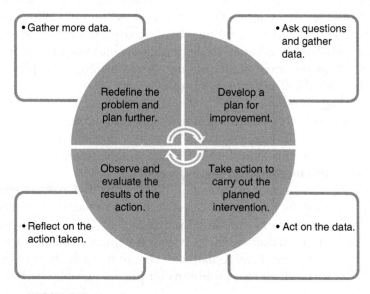

- Gather more data.

- Ask questions and gather data.

Redefine the problem and plan further.

Develop a plan for improvement.

Observe and evaluate the results of the action.

Take action to carry out the planned intervention.

- Reflect on the action taken.

- Act on the data.

FIGURE 5.1 The cyclical nature of action research.

beds. A group consisting of the ED nursing and medical directors, the ED administrator, two ED staff nurses, and one ED physician meets to examine the issue more closely and to write a report based on their examination. Can that research be considered action research if the report based on it is used by the hospital administration to initiate a process that allows better patient flow through the department and the hospital as a whole? The answer is *yes* if the research report is used to initiate change and allows for a follow-up evaluation of the impact of the changes and if those in charge of ED flow are involved in the process. The answer is *no* if the research ended with a report of the investigation sitting on someone's desk or being discussed at a meeting with little or no change in processes. According to Wadsworth (1998), action research is not merely research which it is hoped will be followed by action! It is action which is intentionally researched and modified leading to the next stage of action which is then again intentionally examined for further change and soon is a part of the search itself.

ACTION RESEARCH

The term *action research* was first used in 1946 by Kurt Lewin to describe the process of investigating intergroup relationships and organizational development in the United States (Reason & Rowan, 1981). Action research does not separate the investigation from the action needed to solve the problem. In addition to the traditional handouts and group discussion, action research facilitators use brainstorming, role play, feedback, and critical self-reflection to problem solve (Ferrance, 2000).

According to Meyer (2000), the strength of action research lies in its ability to both generate practical solutions to real-life problems and build capacity among practitioners as they develop and implement activities to solve the identified problem. Action research is a collection of research methodologies used to pursue action (or change) and research (or knowledge) at the same time. Thus, the researchers are directly involved in the practice that is being researched (Ferrance, 2000), and practitioners are directly involved in the research that is being conducted. Action research is based primarily on the assumption that practitioners at immediate and concrete levels are best able to identify, understand, and find solutions for practice problems (Box 5.2).

THE PRINCIPLES OF ACTION RESEARCH

DEMOCRACY
The representative nature of action research may be one of its greatest benefits, as it grounds the research process in real-world practice. Academic researchers and clinical practice experts work together as

BOX 5.2

ASSUMPTIONS UNDERLYING ACTION RESEARCH

Practitioners are best able to understand practice problems in need of a solution.

Change and redirection as needed are essential to action research.

Practice itself is a form of research, as one attempts various ways of obtaining good outcomes.

To be excellent, a practitioner needs to engage in substantial reflection about the nature of practice.

Collaboration among teams of healthcare providers is crucial for process improvement.

equals to determine the problem, the action, its process for change, and the way in which it will be implemented and evaluated (Meyer, 2000). Hierarchal differences are flattened. For example, consider a team of researchers, prison officials, and inmates convened inside a women's maximum security prison to investigate the impact of offering access to higher education to inmates, which ultimately documents that education for prisoners can change communities, reduce crime, and save taxpayer dollars (Torre & Fine, 2006). This is not an easy process. As Prilleltensky (1997) tells us, it is necessary not only to be able to talk about the values of a democratic relationship, but to be able to apply these concepts in action. In the prison study, the inmates had equal voice and participation as did the prison officials. Smith, Bratin, Simone, Chambers, and Chambers (2010) relate the experiences of a gay White male graduate student working on an action research project with inner-city homeless teens who were gay. At the first collaborative meeting, the graduate student was asked to share who he was and why he was there. Despite having discussed this same question with Smith et al., he reflected:

> In the moment that I was asked to participate in that same discussion with participants, I was struck with an anxiety-provoking realization. It was easy to say to my colleagues at school that I wanted to help and advocate for queer youth in our city. However, to say "I want to help you" to a group of people who were actually more comfortable with their sexuality than I was seemed incredibly presumptuous. Immediately, I realized that

I was still not viewing the organization's members as equal partners in the project. (p. 412)

According to Stringer (2007), participation in action research is built upon the key concepts of significant active involvement, performance of specific tasks, support for each other as researchers learn about each other and the problem at hand, setting goals that can be achieved within a certain timeframe, and face-to-face discussion with stakeholders rather than through representatives.

FEEDBACK

Throughout an action research project, findings are given back to participants for validation and to inform decisions about the next stage of the study. This formative style of research is responsive to events as they occur in the field and frequently requires iterations of reflection, action, and re-reflection. Feedback should be information specific, issue focused, and based on observations. The purpose of such feedback is to determine how successful events to improve a process have been and to outline the next steps.

All relevant stakeholders should be provided the necessary feedback on a regular basis. Feedback strategies should be a part of the overall approach to the project and can include regularly scheduled meetings, prearranged visits, telephone calls, or project updates sent by email. According to Stringer (2007), it is important that "each person be linked with others so that participants can discuss their problems, celebrate accomplishments, maintain focus, and sustain their sense of identify with the project" (p. 134).

MULTIPLE GOALS

Action research is characterized by first-, second-, and third-person research goals. In the first person, one's own actions are researched for the purposes of personal change. Second-person research is aimed at ways to improve the group (or community or family). Third-person research is scholarly research aimed primarily at theoretical generalization and/or large-scale change. Goals for each of these agendas are possible within an action research framework. For example, in a research study with the objective of improving the care of older people at risk of delirium, nursing staff wanted experience doing research (first person). They were motivated by the idea of being active participants in developing and implementing improved patient care processes that could reduce the risk of delirium in older people (second person), and they also wanted to evaluate management guidelines and establish quality monitoring criteria for this group of patients (third person; Li et al., 2010).

CHARACTERISTICS OF ACTION RESEARCH

One of the key characteristics that distinguishes action research from most other research approaches, and also constitutes one of its main appeals, is that action research aims at both improving a process and generating knowledge and achieving both at the same time (Kock, 2011). As Meyer (2000) points out, action research "is an approach which demands that participants perceive the need to change and are willing to play an active part in the research and the change process" (p. 178). This level of participation requires a commitment that goes beyond simply collecting data or answering questions. Active participation by stakeholders in the process is crucial to its success. The goals of action research, according to Herr and Anderson (2005), involve generating new knowledge, attaining action-oriented outcomes that are relevant to the setting, and educating team members using a sound research method. To achieve these goals, it is necessary to establish key indicators of performance, which can be used to audit criteria as the project unfolds. Key performance indicators are metrics about how well goals are met. There is no set standard for the development of indicators, but there should be at least one indicator for each project goal. Well-developed indicators are relevant, clearly defined, and easily measured (National Institute for Health and Clinical Excellence [NICE], 2002).

Action research appeals to nurses due to its success in systems improvement and patient outcomes (Badger, 2000) as well as its ability to narrow the theory–practice gap (Rolfe, 1996). Suitable subjects for action research are those that "(a) are real events, which must be managed in real time, (b) provide opportunities for both effective action and learning, and (c) can contribute to the development of theory of what really goes on in hospitals and to the development of nursing knowledge" (Coghlan & Casey, 2001, p. 675). Examples suitable for action research include:

An examination of the use of shared medical equipment
A process to decrease 30-day readmissions among home care patients
The transition from an ICU to a general nursing unit
The development of a procedure for therapeutic hypothermia
A process to address high suicide rates among adolescents

Installation of new computer systems, such as electronic health
   records
Determining the effects of a new teaching strategy

Once the notions of traditional research are swept away, the essential
characteristics of action research are fairly straightforward. Reflection
during each phase of the action cycle is crucial to success. Those involved
must recollect and then critique what has already happened. The
increased understanding that emerges from the reflection is then put
to use in designing the next steps. For example, in the ED waiting- time
study, the action research team first needed to understand the extent and
nature of the waiting-time problem. They began with a general discussion of the issue and how it impacted each of their individual role functions and patient and family satisfaction. Next, they decided they needed
more specific data and set up a process to review the medical records of
those patients who waited longer than 30 minutes in the ED.

FRAMEWORKS FOR ACTION RESEARCH

Action research uses an intentional method that involves (Nursing
Planet, 2011):

- Marking very clear statements about the clinical issue
- Developing goals for improvement
- Formulating action plans to meet the goals
- Observing the effects of the actions
- Reflecting on the observations
- Replanning based on reflections

Yet, the use of various terms to refer to action research (Box 5.1)
implies that the concept of action research has different meanings to
different people, which can lead to very different definitions and forms
of practice (Hinchey, 2008). Dewey (1916), for example, believed that
all research should be done by those central to the issue, rather than
by outsiders. He argued that those in the field needed to do the testing
involved in developing practices. Others, such as Heron (1997), posited
that cooperative inquiry, or collaborative inquiry, is the basis of action
research and that the research is conducted *with* people, rather than
on people. All participants in the process are considered coresearchers.
   Freire believed that action research is participatory and that even
students can participate in research regarding their own learning as

they construct their own knowledge. In what he called PAR, people are empowered to bring change by generating knowledge through reflection on personal experiences and situations (Glasson, Change, & Bidwell, 2008). For example, in a study of palliative care, the practitioner-researchers shared practice stories and analyzed these stories to identify practice issues, such as clinical judgment, the way people die, not being able to provide care, and misunderstandings of palliative nursing (Taylor et al., 2008).

Torbert and Turllen (2004) believed that action inquiry demands attention to what is occurring at the personal, group, and organizational levels in the midst of the action, which allows for immediate learning and understanding of the area being researched.

Kemmis and McTaggart (1988) defined action research as a form of collective inquiry undertaken by participants in social situations to improve their own practice as well as their understanding of those practices and the situations in which these practices are carried out.

The common understanding among these action research frameworks is that real-world practice challenges need analysis and action and reanalysis; the results are shared with the larger community for critique and evaluation; stakeholders are identified early in the process and collectively agree on the problem to be addressed. All participants in an action research project are coresearchers and reflection on the process and results throughout the project is an important action to be taken by all involved.

DATA COLLECTION

Action research primarily draws from qualitative methods of data collection, although the specific method used is dependent upon the question asked and the problem under investigation (Box 5.3). It is important to note that when conducting an action research project, baseline data are needed so that improvement can be documented as a result of action taken. Some of the more common methods used to collect data for an action research study are as follows.

Focus groups, as the name implies, are targeted or focused discussions about issues, actions, or outcomes significant to the research project. Individuals representative of the stakeholders in the project are convened for this interview. Focus groups are useful in developing a more in-depth understanding of a particular issue than could occur at a project meeting with a wide-ranging agenda. Focus group questions can be structured, semistructured, or unstructured,

BOX 5.3

SOME SOURCES OF DATA FOR ACTION RESEARCH

Qualitative
Interviews
Portfolios
Diaries
Field notes
Audiotapes
Photos
Memos
Questionnaires
Focus groups
Anecdotal records
Journals
Individual files
Logs of meetings
Videotapes
Case studies

Quantitative
Surveys
Records
Reports
Self-assessment

depending on the topic for discussion. A researcher might ask only predetermined questions in a structured interview to ensure that the person's specific questions are answered—a useful and efficient strategy when the researcher is clear about exactly needs to be known. However, "less structured interviews hold the possibility of expanding the researcher's thinking; given free rein to shape the conversation, a participant following his own line of thinking may open a new perspective the researcher hadn't considered" (Hinchey, 2008, p. 11). Construction of questions is an important prefocus group activity, as the researcher does not want to influence the participants' answers. For example, the question, "Would you agree that this policy is depriving our staff of needed resources?" calls for a very different response than "Do you have any thoughts on how this policy has affected staff satisfaction?"

Field notes are records written by the researcher about ongoing events that occur during the study. Hinchey (2011) explains that notes can be written in a number of ways, such as sweeping notes (a recording every 5 minutes), event notes (a record of all events that occurred during an observation), critical- incident notes (a recording of crucial points in a study), or summary notes (a summation written at the end of an event or day). Typically, field notes take the form of diary or journal entries, which provide a record of the chronological events and the researcher's reflection on activities and his or her own opinions on the progress of the project.

Surveys are questionnaires used to gather data from many people. Using very focused questions is important with this method. For example, "Do you give medications to your patients daily?" is too broad a question when you want to know the number of medication episodes that occur each day. A free online survey tool, such as Survey Monkey (www.surveymonkey.com), can be effectively used, as these allow for anonymity and multiple question formats.

Documents might need to be reviewed to gain an enhanced understanding of the problem under study. Documents that are important to most process change include meeting minutes, policies, procedures, statistical reports, or quality-improvement (including accreditation) reports. If the action research study is concerned with an education issue, documents, such as student papers, course evaluations, and student handbooks, are also important.

Observation of the processes under study is also common. Observations can be counted (e.g., the number of times a nurse is interrupted when passing medication), measured in time (e.g., the length of time needed to write a bedside report), or described (e.g., the interaction between surgeons and nurses in the operating room). Observation is often combined with interviewing. Interviewing participants can provide a greater understanding of and rationale for activities or behaviors observed. Typically, the observer takes on a passive data-collection role by using a checklist or writing field notes. Audio and video recording may also be used, although this would require additional consideration by the institutional review board and informed consent of participants.

THE CHALLENGES OF ACTION RESEARCH

Action research is not without its challenges. Commitment to the project, which may take a number of months to complete, determination of data ownership, and budget are important issues that need to be discussed in the planning stages of the project.

THE CHALLENGE OF COMMITMENT
The level of commitment required in an action research study goes beyond simply taking part in a meeting, completing a survey, or agreeing to be observed. Core features of action research are that the work happens in the context of active partnership with practitioners. Not only must practitioners see the value of working with researchers, they must want to engage in the research process. Action researchers need to plan for both cycles of action and time for reflection so that practitioners see the value in what they are doing and remain committed (Bradbury, 2010).

THE CHALLENGE OF DEMOCRACY
In action research, participants are equals, as hierarchal differences are flattened (Mendenhall & Doherty, 2005). The researcher works as a facilitator of change, consulting with clinical site practitioners not only on the action process but also on how it will be evaluated, which roots the investigation in everyday practice. Findings are shared and discussed at each stage of the process and used to inform decisions about the next stage. This developmental style of research is thus responsive to naturally occurring clinical events in real time. However, as Meyer (2000) points out, care needs to be taken as the democratic process may be threatening i because it is not a usual feature of healthcare settings. An action researcher needs to be able to work across traditional boundaries (e.g., between health and social work professionals or between hospital and community care settings) and juggle different, sometimes competing, agendas. This requires excellent interpersonal skills as well as research ability. As well, Brown, Bammer, Baltiwala, and Kunreuther (2003) point out, "practitioners bring (their own) frameworks . . . with their own definitions of excellence and effectiveness" (p. 89); therefore researchers need to be aware of the potential need to renegotiate goals (Reed, 2005).

THE CHALLENGE OF PROCESS
Simultaneously gathering and acting on data to influence practice may be a challenge, as this lends itself not only to the discovery of solutions but also to the uncovering of new or unknown clinical issues. It can be a "slow and messy process," especially in the early phases of the research (Mendelhall & Doherty, 2005). Care needs to be taken to remain on target through development of short- and long-term goals and by discussing these at team meetings. In this regard, a project leader skilled in facilitation is needed. Facilitation is a technique in which the actions

of one person make the work of another easier. Facilitation moves along a range of activities that are both task focused (e.g., project management) and enabling (e.g., personal development; Kitson et al., 2008). The facilitator offers change strategies, supports the process, and provides support in the analysis of data. A facilitator needs to be cognizant of the influence of the organizational culture and other influences that may interfere in naturalistic inquiries and to make plans to ease these influences (Holly et al., 2013).

WRITING THE ACTION RESEARCH REPORT

Overall, the final report for an action research study is similar to the standard research report: It contains background information with study purpose, a literature review, and the methods, results, discussion, and conclusions. The additional elements needed in an action research report include:

- A description of the context, which includes descriptions of the organizational structure, stakeholders, and patient served.
- An explanation of how the clinical problem was determined to be a problem in need of action along with the goals of the project and their key indicators of performance.
- A description that focuses on how the clinical problem was investigated prior to the start of the project. Included here should be the viewpoints of those knowledgeable about the clinical problem—using their own words, rather than the usual, more objective research presentation voice—and any available baseline data.
- A description of the role and responsibilities of each of the team members, including the project facilitator.

ACTION RESEARCH VERSUS PAR

Community-based participatory research is action research that involves a community. It is a collaborative approach to research that equitably involves all partners in the research process and recognizes the unique strengths that each brings. Community-based participatory research (CBPR) begins with a research topic of importance to the community with the aim of combining knowledge and action for social change so as to improve community (health; Minkler & Wallerstein, 2003).

Although there are numerous points of convergence between action research and participatory research, one particular difference is the emphasis on collaboration in CBPR. The combination of practice change and collaborative research shifts the emphasis from action and change to collaborative research activities. It is a joint process of knowledge production that leads to new insights on the part of both researchers and practitioners.

CONCLUSIONS

In summary, action research tends to be participative (researchers and clinicians are involved as process partners),cyclic (steps in the process are sequential), qualitative (it deals more with language than numbers); and reflective (the process and results are considered and redefined as needed for the next cycle). See Box 5.4 for a sample of resources used by action researchers.

BOX 5.4

ONLINE RESOURCES FOR ACTION RESEARCH

General Resources
Action Research in the Americas
 http://arnawebsite.org/
Center for Collaborative Action Research
 cadres.pepperdine.edu/ccar
Online Sources for Action Research
 www.lupinworks.com/ar/index.html

For Educators
Action Research in Education
 www.sevenstepswriting.com/samples/action-research-resources/
 www.study.com/academy/lesson/action-research-in-education-examples
-methods-quiz.html

Healthcare
Action Research in Nursing
 www.nursingtimes.net/using-action-research-an-introduction/201088
.article
Carrying Out Action Research on Health Interventions
 https://www.bmj.com/content/347/bmj.f6753

■ QUESTIONS FOR DISCUSSION

1. What is the difference between action research and consulting?
2. How can action research justify its conclusions?
3. Discuss the generalizability of PAR.

■ REFLECTIVE EXERCISE

Reflect on a practice problem that you believe is in need of a solution. Plan your approach:

1. What do you hope to accomplish?
2. What baseline data do you need to fully understand the problem? Where will these data come from?
3. Who will be members of your team?
4. Do you need a champion?
5. Who will you have to convince that change is needed?

EXAMPLES OF ACTION RESEARCH

An Action Research Initiative to Optimize the Well-Being of Older People in Nursing Homes: Challenges and Strategies for Implementing a Complex Intervention

This project was a pilot study using action research to assess strategies that would enable the implementation of a complex intervention approach in nursing homes based on the meaning of screams of older people living with Alzheimer's disease. An action research approach was used with 19 formal and family caregivers from five nursing homes. Clinical nurse specialists and nursing directors were partners (first person). Formal caregivers working in care units where the approach was to be implemented were offered a 7-hour training session. Focus groups and individual interviews were held to assess different implementation strategies (second person). Mitigating strategies in response to the identified challenges were developed. One, for example, was working with formal caregivers to develop and fine-tune tools, including a behavior observation grid and guidelines for establishing partnership with families (third person).

Reference

Bourbonnais, A., Ducharme, F., Landreville, P., Michaud, C., Gauthier, M. A., & Lavallée, M. H. J. (2018). An action research to optimize the well-being of older people in nursing homes: Challenges and strategies for implementing a complex intervention. *Journal of Applied Gerontology*. Epub ahead of print March 1. doi:10.1177/0733464818762068

(continued)

EXAMPLES OF ACTION RESEARCH (*CONTINUED*)

Addressing the Use of Shared Medical Equipment in a Large Urban Hospital
This project addressed the high prevalence of microorganisms, including significant multidrug-resistant microorganisms in the patient care environment. These microorganisms are found in high concentrations on high-touch surfaces such as bedside tables, commodes, over-bed tables, bedrails, doorknobs, sinks and surfaces, and shared noncritical patient equipment. Stringent and frequent decontamination of these surfaces has been shown to prevent transmission and curtail outbreaks. This project aimed to construct and implement a best practice approach for the use and disinfection of noncritical portable medical devices to decrease equipment-related HAIs (hospital-acquired infections). The most common portable equipment (glucometers and portable temperature units) were targeted. Using action research with pre- and postintervention observation and focus groups, the community of practice consisted of two nurse managers, the director of education, the director of infection control, and a nursing faculty member. The director of education served as the group facilitator to guide the team through identification and understanding of evidence, while the faculty member provided guidance in the scientific method (first person). The project was conducted on two inpatient units: a neonatal intensive care unit and an adult medical–surgical unit in a large urban medical center. Focus groups were held to determine current practice and identify barriers to the cleaning of shared noncritical patient equipment. Participants in the focus groups were the clinical staff providing patient care within these units who had first identified the issue, that is, the professional nurses and nursing assistants and staff from environmental services (second person). Baseline data for multidrug-resistant HAI rates for the medical–surgical and neonatal intensive care unit were obtained. Observations were conducted by the infection control practitioners using an observational data tool to determine how and if staff members were cleaning equipment between patient use and according to the manufacturer's recommendations. Adapting evidence to the local context, examining context for barriers to implementation, and developing a local plan of action to put evidence into action were major steps. A three-point plan was developed: education, policy and procedure revision, and a change in the location of disinfection supplies (second person).

Preinterventional data collection revealed equipment was not cleaned per the manufacturer's recommendations 40.54% of the time, users could not identify whether equipment was clean 13.51% of the time, and equipment was visibly soiled 16.21% of the time. Postinterventional data collection revealed that users cleaned the equipment both before and after using it 69.2% of the time. These findings were significant at less than $p = 0.05$. When equipment was cleaned, the correct cleaning agent was used according to the manufacturer's instructions 100% of the time. When equipment was not cleaned, sanitizing solutions were not available 50% of the time. One of the greatest contributors to staff not cleaning equipment, identified during the focus group sessions, was that sanitizing solutions were not readily available. In every instance staff identified the importance of cleaning equipment in between each patient use, demonstrating that there was not a lack of knowledge in this area. The lack of knowledge was that staff

(continued)

EXAMPLES OF ACTION RESEARCH (*CONTINUED*)

could not always identify the manufacturer's recommendations for proper cleaning of equipment. This was addressed by having a representative of the solution company conduct training sessions on the use of the solution. Given the positive results of this action study in the identification and resolution of a clinical issue identified by frontline staff, the project will be implemented in all areas of the medical center (third person).

Reference

Bugel, M. J., & Scuderi, D. (2011). *Addressing the use of shared medical equipment in a large urban hospital.* In C. Holly (Ed.), *Scholarly inquiry and the DNP capstone* (pp. 46–48). New York, NY: Springer Publishing.

■ SUGGESTED READINGS

Brownhill, S., Ungarova, T., & Bipazhanova, A. (2017). Jumping the first hurdle: Framing action research question using the ice cream cone model. *Methodological Innovations, 10*(3), 1–11. doi:10.1177/2059799117741407

Casey, M., O'Leary, D., & Coghlan, D. (2018). Unpacking action research and implementation science: Implications for nursing. *Journal of Advanced Nursing, 74*(5), 1051–1058. doi:10.1111/jan.13494

MacLennon, H. (2018). Student perceptions of plagiarism avoidance competencies: An action research case study. *Journal of the Scholarship of Teaching and Learning, 18*(1), 58–74. doi:10.14434/josotl.v18i1.22350

■ REFERENCES

Aylward, P., Murphy, P., Colmer, K., & O'Neill, M. (2010). Findings from an evaluation of an intervention targeting Australian parents of young children with attachment issues: The "Through the Looking Glass" (TtLG) project. *Australasian Journal of Early Childhood, 35*(3), 14–24.

Badger, T. G. (2000). Action research, change and methodological rigour. *Journal of Nursing Management, 8*, 201–207. doi:10.1046/j.1365-2834.2000.00174.x

Bourbonnais, A., Ducharme, F., Landreville, P., Michaud, C., Gauthier, M. A., & Lavallée, M. H. J. (2018). An action research to optimize the well-being of older people in nursing homes: Challenges and strategies for implementing a complex intervention. *Journal of Applied Gerontology*. Epub ahead of print March 1. doi:10.1177/0733464818762068

Bradbury, H. H. (2010). What is good action research. *Action Research, 8*(1), 93–109. doi:10.1177/1476750310362435

Brown, D. L., Bammer, G., Baltiwala, S., & Kunreuther, F. (2003). Framing practice-research engagement for democratizing knowledge. *Action Research, 1*, 81–102. doi:10.1177/14767503030011006

Bugel, M. J., & Scuderi, D. (2011). *Addressing the use of shared medical equipment in a large urban hospital.* In C. Holly (Ed.), *Scholarly inquiry and the DNP capstone* (pp. 46–48). New York, NY: Springer Publishing.

Coghlan, D., & Casey, M. (2001). Action research from the inside: Issues and challenges in doing action research in your own hospital. *Journal of Advanced Nursing, 35*(5), 674–682.

Dewey, J. (1916). *Democracy and education: An introduction to the philosophy of education.* New York, NY: Macmillan.

Ferrance, E. (2000). *Themes in education: Action research.* Providence, RI: Northeast and Regional Educational Laboratory at Brown University.

Glasson, J., Chang, E., & Bidewell J. (2008). The value of participatory action research in clinical nursing practice. International *Journal of Nursing Practice, 14*(1), 34–39.

Heron, J. (1997). *Co-operative inquiry: Research into the human condition.* Thousand Oaks, CA: Sage.

Herr, K., & Anderson, G. L. (2005). *The action research dissertation.* Thousand Oaks, CA: Sage.

Hinchey, P. (2008). *Action research primer.* New York, NY: Peter Lang Publishing.

Holly, C., Percy, M., Salmond, S., Caldwell, B., Echevarria, M., & Bugel, M. J. (2013). *When cultures collide: Academic and clinical teams join forces to move evidence into practice.* Newark, NJ: University of Medicine and Dentistry of NJ, School of Nursing.

Kemmis, S., & McTaggart, R. (Eds.). (1988). *The action research planner* (3rd ed.). Waurn Ponds, VIC: Deakin University Press.

Kitson, A., Rycroft-Malone, J., Harvey, G., McCormack, B., Seers, K., & Titchen, A. (2008). Evaluating the successful implementation of evidence into practice using the PARIHS Framework: Theoretical and practical challenges. *Implementation Science, 3*(1), 913–924. Retrieved from http://www.implementationscience.com/content/3/1/1

Kock, N. (2011): Action research: Its nature and relationship to human-computer interaction. In M. Soegaard & R. F. Dam (Eds.), *Encyclopedia of human-computer interaction.* Copenhagen, DK: The Interaction Design Foundation. Retrieved from http://www.interactiondesign.org/encyclopedia/action_research.html

Li, P., Bashford, L., Schwarger, G., Spain, R., Ryan, H., Oakman, M., . . . Higgins, I. (2010). Clinicians experience of participating in an action research study. *Contemporary Nurse, 35*(2), 147–156. doi:10.5172/conu.2010.35.2.147

Mendenhall, T., & Doherty, W. (2005). Action research methods in family therapy. In F. Piercy & D. Sprenkle (Eds.), *Research methods in family therapy* (2nd ed., pp. 100–117). New York, NY: Guilford Press.

Meyer, J. (2000). Using qualitative methods in health related action research. *BMJ, 32*(06), 178. doi:10.1136/bmj.320.7228.178

Minkler, M., & Wallerstein, N. (2003). *Community-based participatory research for health.* San Francisco, CA: Jossey-Bass .

National Institute for Health and Clinical Excellence. (2002). *Principles for best practice in clinical audit.* Oxford, England: Radical Medical Press.

Nursing Planet. (2011). *Action research in nursing.* Retrieved from http://nursingplanet.com/Nursing_Research/action_research_nursing.html

Prilleltensky, I. (1997). Values, assumptions, and practices: Assessing the moral implications of psychological discourse and action. *American Psychologist, 52*(5), 517–535.

Reason, P., & Bradbury, H. (2007). *Handbook of action research* (2nd ed.). London, England: Sage.

Reason, P., & Rowan, J. (1981). *Human inquiry: A sourcebook for paradigm research.* Chichester, England: Wiley.

Reed, J. (2005). Using action research in nursing practice with older people: Democratizing knowledge. *Journal of Clinical Nursing, 14*(5), 594–600. doi:10.1111/j.1365-2702.2005.01110.x

Rolfe, G. (1996). Going to extremes: Action research, grounded practice and the theory–practice gap in nursing. *Journal of Advanced Nursing, 24,* 1315–1320. doi:10.1111/j.1365-2648.1996.tb01040.x

Smith, L., Bratin, L., Simone, D., Chambers, D., & Chambers, S. (2010). Between idealism and reality: Meeting the challenges of participatory action research. *Action Research, 8*(4), 407–425.

Stringer, E. (2007). *Action research* (3rd ed.). Thousand Oaks, CA: Sage.

Torbert, W., & Turllen, J. (2004). First-, second-, and third-person research in practice. *Systems Thinker, 15*(1), 7–8.

Torre, M., & Fine, M. (2006). Researching and resisting: Democratic policy research by and for youth. In S. Ginwright, P. Noguera, & J. Cammarota (Eds.), *Beyond resistance! Youth activism and community change: New democratic possibilities for practice and policy for America's youth* (pp. 269–285). New York, NY: Routledge.

Wadsworth, Y. (1998). What is participatory action research? *Action Research International*, Paper 2. Retrieved from http://www.scu.edu.au/schools/gcm/ar/ari/p-ywadsworth98.html

CHAPTER 6

Case Study Research

■ OBJECTIVES

At the end of this chapter, you will be able to:

- Describe the key features of a case study.
- Explain the components of a case study.
- Explain the strategies for making meaning from case study data.
- Apply the criteria for selecting a case for study of a clinical problem.

■ KEY CONCEPTS

- Case study projects bring a greater depth of understanding to complex issues through contextual analysis.
- A case study can focus on an individual, a group (such as a family or hospital unit), an institution, or an entire community.
- Case study methodology is appropriate for describing, exploring, and understanding a phenomenon in its real-life context.
- A variety of data-collection methods are used in case studies.
- Case study research fits within the postpositive philosophy, meaning that there is thinking and reflection on what resulted after it happened.

INTRODUCTION

A case study begins with a story. The story is followed by an intensive analysis. Constructing a case study is an opportunity to highlight success, to bring attention to a particular challenge or difficulty, or to describe a unique or unusual event. Cases might be selected because they are highly effective, not ineffective, representative, typical, or of special interest (Zucker, 2001). A case study also promotes an inquiry method that allows investigation of a clinical problem within a context bounded by time, place, and activity and in which multiple sources of evidence are used (Yin, 2004).

As a project method, a case study can be used when the interaction among many factors needs to be understood. Case studies have been criticized as being unreliable and nongeneralizable as the number of cases studied is usually very small; in fact, one case can make a case study. On the other hand, a case study describes real-life situations, issues, and problems and provides an understanding as to how clinicians resolve issues or develop programs. "Thus, case studies comprise more detail, richness, completeness, and variance—that is, depth than other types of methods" (Flyvbjerg, 2011, p. 301). The value of the case study lies in its invaluable descriptions of processes, interactions, and relationships. "Such descriptions are phenomenologically distinctive and permit identification with the experience of the worker and the reality of the clinical encounter, albeit vicariously" (Brandell & Varkas, 2001, p. 294).

The terms *case study*, *case review*, and *case report* are used synonymously; however, the key feature of a case study is that it is idiographic, meaning that the unit of study (or unit of analysis) is a single unit, and the unit can be an individual, population, team, family, community, organization, or process (Brandell & Varkas, 2001). A case study is a "systematic inquiry into an event or a set of related events which aims to describe and explain the phenomenon of interest" (Bromley, 1990, p. 302), with a defined focus and a specific time frame (Miles, Huberman, & Saldana, 2014). A case study allows a deeper understanding of a complex issue or process and can add to what is already known. This is accomplished through a detailed contextual analysis of events or conditions and their relationships using documentation, archival records, interviews, direct observations, participant observation, and physical artifacts among other data-collection methods (Yin, 2009; Zucker, 2001). For example, case studies of individual patients often involve in-depth interviews with participants and key informants, review of the medical records, observation, and excerpts from patients' personal writings and diaries, whereas case studies of an organization or system involve review of meeting agenda and minutes, reports, policies, and procedures. Woodside (2010) maintains that using multiple methods such as these to triangulate data confirms and deepens understanding, providing what Yin (2009) calls *a chain of evidence*.

A case study done for the purpose of examining phenomena is not the same as a case study used for teaching purposes in the classroom. Freud's case study of Dora is a famous example of the use of a case study to explain unusual symptoms that might be useful in similar situations (Freud, 1963). Teaching case studies, such as Freud's example, which focus on application of theory, are not concerned with rigor or empirical data (Yin, 2009). Conducting case study research implies that you have a question to explore and will use the scientific method to find an answer.

According to Yin (2009), a case study design should be used when (a) the question guiding the study is a *how* and/or a *why* question, (b) the behavior of those involved in the study cannot be manipulated, (c) the context is important to the study, or (d) there are no clear boundaries between the unit of analysis and the context.

TYPES OF CASE STUDIES

Case studies can be exploratory, explanatory, or descriptive (Yin, 2009). Description in a case study attempts to answer the *who, what, where, when*, and *how* questions. Explanation attempts to answer the *why* question. Prediction in case study research includes forecasting near-term and/or long-term behaviors or events (Woodside, 2010). Any of the three can use single or multiple cases. Single cases are used to characterize a unique or rare case. Single-case studies are also ideal for cases in which an observer may have access to a phenomenon that was previously inaccessible. These studies can be holistic or embedded. An embedded case involves more than one unit of analysis in the same case study. Multiple-case studies are repetitive; that is, each individual case study is unique and could stand alone as a single case, but together they form a more powerful representation of the whole, as, for example, in Kitson et al.'s (2015) study of the process of facilitation to support quality-improvement efforts.

Exploratory case studies are used to explore those situations in which the intervention being evaluated has no clear, single set of outcomes (Yin, 2009). Often, exploratory case studies are undertaken prior to beginning primary or discovery research to develop hypotheses. Flugman, Perin, and Spiegel (2003), for example, documented reports of numbers of adolescents taking adult education courses and characteristics of youth in comparison with those of older students and to investigate additional issues and questions, such as characteristics of adult education programs serving youth.

Explanatory case studies describe suspected relationships that are too complex for survey research and attempt to link a program\imple-mentation with its effects. This type of case study looks for relation-ships among variables or causes for specific outcomes. For example, using a case study approach, Horigan, Rocchiccioli, and Trimm (2012) explained the relationships among chronic kidney disease (CKD), renal pathology, and renal fatigue in a 33-year-old woman on dialysis.

Descriptive case studies provide a detailed profile of a subject, an intervention, or a phenomenon within a real-life context. A classic example is the case report study of five homosexual males who devel-oped a rare pneumonia. This case study led to the subsequent discovery of AIDS/HIV. The initial cases involved a cluster of injection drug users and gay men with no known cause of impaired immunity who exhibited symptoms of *Pneumocystis carinii* pneumonia (PCP), a rare opportun-istic infection known to occur in people with compromised immune systems (Friedman-Kien, 1981; Hymes et al., 1981).

COMPONENTS OF A CASE STUDY

Yin (1994) identified five components that are important for case studies:

- A study's questions
- Its propositions, if any
- Its unit(s) of analysis
- The logic linking the data to the propositions
- The criteria for interpreting the findings

Case study *questions* are phrased as a *how* or a *why* question. For exam-ple, Lo (2002) wanted to know how nursing students coped with stress over the course of a 3-year nursing program.

The study's *propositions* focus on the aims of the study and allow for what data to collect. Propositions are derived from theories, literature, experience, or empirical data and provide a framework for the case study. An exploratory case study, however, may not have propositions; rather it will have a stated purpose or hunch as it seeks to explore the phenome-non as a prelude to primary research. The more a study contains specific propositions, the more it will stay within its aims and time frame.

Examples of propositions from the research literature are:

- Some women may choose not to have reconstructive surgery fol-lowing mastectomy due to a fear of pain (Wallace, Wallace, Lee, & Dobke, 1996).

■ For hospitals in which the elective surgery caseload is limited by nursing recruitment, to increase one surgeon's operating room time either another surgeon's time must be decreased, the nurses need to be paid a premium for working longer hours, or higher priced travel nurses can be contracted (Dexter, Blake, Penning, & Lubarsky, 2002).

The *unit of analysis* is a critical factor in case study research. To determine the specific unit of analysis in a case study, ask the following questions:

■ Do I want to understand something about individuals?
■ Do I want to evaluate a program?
■ Do I want to understand a process?
■ Do I want to compare differences between groups or organizations?

According to Flyvbjerg (2011), if you choose to do a case study, the choice is less about what method to use, than what is to be studied. The individual unit may be studied in a number of ways, for instance, qualitatively or quantitatively, analytically or hermeneutically, or by mixed methods. There may be more than one unit of analysis in a case study. For example, if you decide to analyze student performance based on a new curriculum, the student is the unit of analysis. However, you might also want to explore how the teacher taught the class and the classroom environment. In this case, the unit of analysis is actually the group, the teacher, and the classroom environment.

Linking the data to *propositions* and the *criteria for interpreting* the findings are the least developed aspects of case studies (Yin, 1994). The challenge is to reduce the volume of data collected within the context of the propositions and framework developed for the study. Pattern matching offers some solutions. This technique compares an empirically derived pattern with a predicted one. If the patterns match, the internal reliability of the study is enhanced. Explanation building is considered a form of pattern matching, in which the analysis of the case study is carried out by building an explanation of the case. This implies that it is most useful in explanatory case studies, but it is possible to use explanation building for exploratory cases as well as part of a hypothesis-generating process. Explanation building is an iterative process that begins with a theoretical statement, refines it, revises the proposition, and repeats this process continually until no further explanation can be determined (Tellis, 1997a, 1997b).

DEALING WITH VALIDITY AND RELIABILITY

Validity and reliability need special attention in case study research. Construct validity is problematic in case study research due to the high potential of investigator subjectivity. Yin (1994, 2009) proposed three remedies to counteract this: using multiple sources of evidence, establishing a chain of evidence, and having a draft of the case study report reviewed by key informants (member checking).

Internal validity is a concern only in explanatory cases. This is usually a problem of interpretation in case studies and can be dealt with using pattern matching, which has been described earlier.

External validity deals with knowing whether the results are generalizable beyond the immediate case; the more variations in places, people, and procedures a case study can withstand and still yield the same findings, the more external validity it has. An exacting literature review helps ensure external validity.

Reliability refers to the stability, accuracy, and precision of measurement. Reliability is achieved in many ways in a case study. One of the most important methods of achieveing reliability is through the development of the case study protocol. A case study protocol contains the procedures and general rules that will be followed when constructing the case. A typical protocol should have the following sections:

- An overview of the case study project (objectives, issues, rationale for a case study approach, topics being investigated)
- Field procedures (how sites will be accessed, what sources of information will be sought)
- Case study questions (specific questions that guide data collection)
- An outline of the final case report (Yin, 1994, p. 64)

COLLECTING CASE STUDY DATA

There are six primary sources of evidence used in case study research:

1. Documents
2. Archival records
3. Interviews (open ended or focused; surveys are also used)
4. Direct observation (formal or casual)
5. Participant observation
6. Physical artifacts

Not all sources of data are necessary for every case study. Each case requires a unique set of data to be collected. Documents could be letters, memoranda, agendas, meeting minutes, policies, procedures, newspaper articles, or any document that is relevant to the case. The documents serve to corroborate the evidence from other sources. Documents are also useful for making inferences about events. Documents are also communications between parties involved in the study.

Archival documents can be service records, organizational records, organizational charts, lists of names, survey data, maps, and other such records. The investigator has to be careful in evaluating the accuracy of the records before using them. Even if the records are quantitative, they might still not be accurate.

Interviews are one of the most important sources of case study information. They can be either open ended, focused, structured, or episodic. In an open-ended interview, key respondents are asked to comment about certain events. They may propose solutions or provide insight into events. They may also corroborate evidence obtained from other sources. It is necessary to interview more than one informant to avoid becoming dependent on a single source of information. The focused interview uses an informal set of questions when it is necessary to determine the authenticity of data collected elsewhere. A more planned interview uses a more detailed set of questions, called an interview schedule. These questions are predetermined and very specific. Field observation may also be used to corroborate data collected for use in a case study. Use of more than one method of collecting data enhances the validity of collected data.

Direct observation occurs when a field visit is conducted during the case study. It could be as simple as casual data-collection activities or formal protocols used to measure and record behaviors. This technique is useful for providing additional information about the topic being studied. Authenticity of collected data is enhanced when more than one observer is used. Observation provides access to what people actually do in a situation, rather than what they have written or explained. In doing an observation, watching what people do and say is called *detached observation*. For example, if the case study involves the elderly with communication or mobility difficulties, then observation is going to be more productive than interviews (Gillham, 2010). Participant observation provides the researcher a unique opportunity to study phenomena or activities as they occur; however, care must be taken not to interfere with the usual course of events.

Physical artifacts can be tools, instruments, samples of students' work, journals, or some other physical evidence that may be collected during the study as part of a field visit. The perspective of the researcher can be broadened as a result of the discovery.

ANALYZING CASE STUDY EVIDENCE

When analyzing results for a case study, opinion tends to count more than statistical methods. The usual idea is to try and collate your data into a manageable form and construct a narrative around it. Miles et al. (2014) suggested analytic techniques such as rearranging the arrays; placing the evidence in a matrix of categories; creating flowcharts or data displays; tabulating the frequency of different events; and using means, variances, and cross-tabulations to examine the relationships between variables.

First, an analytic strategy must be used that will lead to conclusions. Yin (1994) presented two strategies for general use: One is to rely on theoretical propositions of the study and then to analyze the evidence based on those propositions.

Pattern matching is another major mode of analysis. This type of logic compares an empirical pattern with a predicted one.

Yin (1994) encouraged researchers to make every effort to produce an analysis of the highest quality. In order to accomplish this, he presented four principles that should attract the researcher's attention:

- Show that the analysis relied on all the relevant evidence.
- Include all major rival interpretations in the analysis.
- Address the most significant aspect of the case study.
- Use prior expert knowledge to further the analysis.

There are some valuable sources of information that offer guidance for case study methodologies. Stake (1995) and Yin (1994, 2009) have provided specific guidelines for the development of the design and execution of a case study.

1. *Form a question and determine the objectives for the case study.*

As with all research, case study research begins with the formulation of a question, and particular to case studies, the setting of boundaries. For example, statistical analysis may have shown that maternal and infant mortality in some African countries is increasing. A case study can be a powerful and focused tool for determining the social and economic pressures driving this. However, can you study both infant and maternal mortality in a reasonable time frame? What country (ies) would be the focus?

To assist in framing the question, researchers conduct a literature review. This review establishes what research has been conducted previously and leads to refined, insightful questions about the problem (Zucker, 2001). A precise question can identify the key words to use in the literature search, the methods of data collection to use, and the method of analysis to be used in the study.

REPORTING THE CASE STUDY

Case studies frequently contain a strong element of narrative about a sequence of events and their relationship to each other and to the context (Flyvbjerg, 2011). Examples of what you have found or observed are useful but should be only a brief narrative; numerical data should be used judiciously (see Box 6.1).

The use of narrative involves the danger, however, of committing what has been called *the narrative fallacy* (Flyvbjerg, 2011). This fallacy consists of a human propensity to simplify data through a predilection for compact stories over complex data sets. It is easier for the human mind to remember and make decisions on the basis of stories with meaning than it is to remember strings of data. This is one reason why narrative case studies are so powerful and why many of the classics in case study research are written in narrative format. But humans read meaning into

BOX 6.1

SUGGESTED OUTLINE FOR PRESENTING CASE STUDIES

1. The problem
   a. Identify the problem.
   b. Explain why the problem is important.
   c. How was the problem identified?
   d. Was the process for identifying the problem effective?
2. Steps taken to address the problem
3. Results
4. Challenges and how they were met
5. Beyond results
6. Lessons learned

data and also compose stories, even when this is unwarranted. In case study research, the way to avoid the narrative fallacy is no different than the way of avoiding other errors: Consistently check for validity and reliability in how data are collected, analyzed, and presented.

Writing a case study research report is a challenge because it involves using a variety of evidence gathered in different ways, skill is required to weave this evidence into a coherent narrative, and one also needs to maintain the focus and direction determined by the study's aims and specific research questions (Graham, 2010). A case study should report findings so that the reader can reach the same understanding as the researcher (Zucker, 2001).

CONCLUSIONS

Case studies are complex because they generally involve multiple sources of data, may include multiple cases within a study, and produce large amounts of data for analysis. Researchers from many disciplines use the case study method to build upon theory, to produce new theory, to dispute or challenge theory, to explain a situation, to provide a basis to apply solutions to situations, to explore, or to describe an object or phenomenon. The advantages of the case study method are its applicability to real-life contemporary human situations and its public accessibility through written reports. Case study results relate directly to the everyday experience and facilitate an understanding of complex real-life situations.

The goal of the case study method is to provide the most accurate description possible given the available data. Miles et al. (2014) have described 13 strategies for generating meaning from qualitative data. Such tactics range from descriptive to explanatory and from concrete to abstract. According to Miles et al., the first three tactics tell us "what goes with what." The next two tell us "what's there." The next two help "sharpen our understanding." The next four help us "see things and their relationships more abstractly." Finally the last two help us to "assemble a coherent understanding of the data" (pp. 245–246).

■ QUESTIONS FOR DISCUSSION

1. How can case studies inform or advance degree of nursing practice (DNP)?
2. Read the following case study:

Stelter R. (2015). I tried so many diets, now I want to do it differently—A single case study on coaching for weight loss. *International Journal of Qualitative Studies on Health and Well-being, 10,* 26925. doi:10.3402/qhw.v10.26925

- In your initial reading, some of the case's facts, elements, or issues may not have seemed very important or transparent. Why do you think they were included?
- As you reflect on the case, are there items that have grown in importance in your mind that need greater clarity?
- What areas need clarification?
- What thoughts do you have after reading the case study?

■ REFLECTIVE EXERCISE

Identify a topic that you would like to study, for example, "How is the process of nurses' bedside reporting going?" or "What nonpharmacological methods work best to prevent acute delirium in the ICU patient?" Answer the following questions:

- Why would this be a case study?
- What criteria did you use for selecting this case?
- What case study approach would work best?
- What is the unit of analysis?
- What are one or two propositions underlying the question? What is the source of the propositions?
- What data would I need to collect to answer the question?
- What will I do with the findings of the study?
- How will the findings inform or change clinical practice?

EXAMPLES OF CASE STUDY PROJECTS

A Case Study of the Implementation of an Electronic Health Record in Preadmission Units and Day Surgery Centers
The purpose of this project was to construct a case study on the implementation of an electronic health record (EHR) in a preadmission unit and day surgery center. Following Yin's (1994) recommendation that specific

(continued)

EXAMPLES OF CASE STUDY PROJECTS (*CONTINUED*)

questions guide the investigator during data collection, the research questions guiding the study were:

1. How is a technological innovation diffused on nursing units?
2. How do staff influence success of the diffusion?
3. What are the facilitators and barriers to implementation of new technology?

Data were collected using document review, observation (time and motion study), stakeholder interview, and a survey of nurses' attitudes about the use of computers. There were no statistically significant findings on the paired samples t-test comparing pre– and post–mean scores on the nurses' attitudes toward computers scale ($t = 1.938$, $p = .094$ [sig. 2-tailed]). However, comparing the preimplementation and postimplementation mean scores revealed that nurses had more negative attitudes postcomputerization as evidenced by a decreased mean attitude score from 2.53 to 1.78. An interview provided more in-depth analysis to understand this finding. Overall, the nurses preferred the EHR to paper records, but wanted it to better support their nursing practice. A content analysis of open-ended questions about perceived facilitators and barriers provided similar results. Perceived facilitators frequently encountered by nurses with the EHRs were as follows: easy to use, accessibley, legibile, saves time, provides continuity of care, and improves quality of patient care. Perceived barriers and problems with the current EHRs were as follows: not enough time, frequent computer freezing, unfamiliarity/computer anxiety, privacy/Health Insurance Portability and Accountability Act (HIPAA), time-consuming to use, lack of eye contact. A time and motion study was included as a collection method in the case study research to assess the amount of time nurses spend for documentation. Initially, results showed that EHR documentation time took 2.5 minutes longer than the paper chart documentation time. It was expected that more time would be used for documenting electronically because of the added facility-defined features such as mandatory fields to improve regulatory compliance and enhancement of screens/forms to include nationally recognized instruments of evidence-based practice(e.g., Braden scale and pain assessment scale). There were variables, such as interruptions, lack of computer skills, and inefficient time use, that affect nursing workflow. If the workflow process could be streamlined and inefficient time use eliminated or reduced, the hospital could generate an annual cost savings of approximately $119, 891. Initially, there was some resistance from the staff due to the change from paper to electronic documentation and some technical difficulties, but with the training, support, and follow-up provided, the staff were able to recognize the value of the system. Considerations for users' needs and preferences and administrative support are essential to promote EHR adoption. Results of this case study will be valuable to help streamline EHRs and improve/redesign nursing workflow as well as to develop effective implementation strategies in the diffusion of the EHR hospital wide. It was evident that the design enhancements and implementation processes

(continued)

EXAMPLES OF CASE STUDY PROJECTS (*CONTINUED*)

would be very important in fostering staff attitudes and improving workflow performance.

References

Estrada, R. (2011). Case study research. In C. Holly (Ed.), *Scholarly inquiry and the DNP capstone* (pp. 49–68). New York, NY: Springer Publishing.

Yin, R. (1994). *Case study research: Design and methods* (2nd ed.). Beverly Hills, CA: Sage.

PATTERNS OF COMMUNITY PARTICIPATION ACROSS THE SEASONS: A YEAR-LONG CASE STUDY OF THREE CANADIAN WHEELCHAIR USERS

This case study explored patterns of wheelchair users' community participation given differences in weather conditions. Using a gobal positioning system (GPS), data were collected for 1 week per month across 1 year. An interview was conducted with the three participants once per month to gain a better understanding of their participation within their communities. Three distinct patterns were identified in response to variations in weather conditions: (1) season and transportation are linked: winter limits community participation; (2) winter conditions are surmountable; and (3) winter conditions affect ease, choice, and options, but not overall participation. It was concluded that although winter weather conditions pose a challenge, ready access to vehicular transportation that is accessible regardless of weather conditions is a key factor in promoting community participation across the year for wheelchair users.

Reference

Ripat, J., Borisoff, J. F., Grant, L. E., & Chan, F. H. N. (2018). Patterns of community participation across the seasons: A year-long case study of three Canadian wheelchair users. *Disability and Rehabilitation, 40*(6), 722–731. doi:10.1080/09638288.2016.1271463

■ SUGGESTED READINGS

Baxter, P., & Jack, S. (2008). Qualitative case study methodology: Study design and implementation for novice researchers. *Qualitative Report, 13*(4), 544–559. Retrieved from http://www.nova.edu/ssss/QR/QR13-4/baxter.pdf

Cronin, C. (2014). Using case study research as a rigorous form of inquiry. *Nursing Research, 21*(5), 19–27. doi:10.7748/nr.21.5.19.e1240

Hyett, N., Kenny, A., & Dickson-Swift, V. (2014). Methodology or method? A critical review of qualitative case study reports. *International Journal of Qualitative Studies on Health and Well-Being*, 9, 23606. doi:10.3402/qhw.v9.23606

Taylor, R., & Thomas-Gregory, A. (2015). Case study research. *Nursing Standard*, 29(41), 36–40. doi:10.7748/ns.29.41.36.e8856

■ REFERENCES

Brandell, J., & Varkas, T. (2001). Narrative case studies. In B. A. Thyer (Ed.), *The handbook of social work research methods* (pp. 293–307). Thousand Oak, CA: Sage.

Bromley, D. B. (1990). Academic contributions to psychological counselling: I. A philosophy of science for the study of individual cases. *Counselling Psychology Quarterly*, 3(3), 299–307. doi:10.1080/09515079008254261

Dexter, F., Blake, J., Penning, D. H., & Lubarsky, D. (2002). Calculating a potential increase in hospital margin for elective surgery by changing operating room time allocations or increasing nursing staffing to permit completion of more cases: A case study. *Anesthesia and Analgesia*, 94(1), 138–142. doi:10.1213/00000539-200201000-00026

Estrada, R. (2011). Case study research. In C. Holly (Ed.), *Scholarly inquiry and the DNP capstone*. New York, NY: Springer Publishing.

Flugman, B., Perin, D., & Spiegel, S. (2003). *An exploratory case study of 16-20 year old students in adult education programs*. New York, NY: Center for advanced study in education, City University of New York. Retrieved from http://web.gc.cuny.edu/dept/case/adult_ed/Adult_Ed_TimesRoman_Final_Rpt.pdf

Flyvbjerg, B. (2011). Case study. In N. K. Denzin and Y. S. Lincoln (Eds.), *The Sage handbook of qualitative research* (4th ed., pp. 311–313). Thousand Oaks, CA: Sage.

Freud, S. (1963). *Dora: An analysis of a case of hysteria*. New York, NY: Simon & Schuster.

Friedman-Kien, A. E. (1981). Disseminated Kaposi's sarcoma syndrome in young homosexual men. *Journal of the American Academy of Dermatology*, 5(4), 468–471. doi:10.1016/S0190-9622(81)80010-2

Gillham, B. (2010). *Case study research methods*. London, England: Continuum.

Graham, B. (2010). *Case study research methods*. New York, NY: Bloomsbury Publishing.

Horigan, A., Rocchiccioli, J., & Trimm, D. (2012). Dialysis and fatigue: Implications for nurses—A case study analysis. *MEDSURG Nursing*, 21(3), 158–175.

Hymes, K. B., Cheung, T., Greene, J. B., Prose, N. S., Marcus, A., Ballard, H., . . . Laubenstein, L. J. (1981). Kaposi's sarcoma in homosexual men—A report of eight cases. *Lancet*, 2(8247), 598–600. doi:10.1016/S0140-6736(81)92740-9

Kitson, A. L., Wiechula, R., Conroy, T., Whitaker, N., Holly, C., & Salmond, S. (2015). Case study of the Signature project—An Australian–US knowledge translation project. In G. Harvey & A. Kitson (Eds.), *Implementing evidence-based practice in healthcare: A facilitation guide* (pp. 185–204). Abingdon, UK: Routledge.

Lo, R. (2002). A longitudinal study of perceived level of stress, coping and self-esteem of undergraduate nursing students: An Australian case study. *Journal of Advanced Nursing*, 39(2), 119–126. doi:10.1046/j.1365-2648.2000.02251.x

Miles, M., Huberman, A. M., & Saldana, J. (2014). *Qualitative data analysis* (3rd ed.). Thousand Oaks, CA: Sage.

Stake, R. E. (1995). *The art of case study research*. Thousand Oaks, CA: Sage.

Tellis, W. (1997a). Application of case study methodology. *Qualitative Report*, 3(2). Retrieved from http://www.nova.edu/ssss/QR/QR3-3/tellis2.html

Tellis, W. (1997b). Introduction to case study. *Qualitative Report*, 3(2). Retrieved from http://www.nova.edu/ssss/QR/QR3-2/tellis1.html

Wallace, M. S., Wallace, A. M., Lee, J., & Dobke, M. K. (1996). Pain after breast surgery: A survey of 282 women. *Pain, 66*(2–3), 195–205. doi:10.1016/0304-3959(96)03064-3

Woodside, A. (2010). Building theory from case study. In Woodside, A. (Ed.), *Case study research: Theory, methods, practice* (p. 1). Bingley, UK: Emerald Publishing Group.

Yin, R. (1994). *Case study research: Design and methods* (2nd ed.). Beverly Hills, CA: Sage.

Yin, R. (2009). *Case study research: Design and methods* (4th ed.). Beverly Hills, CA: Sage.

Zucker, D. M. (2001). Using case study methodology in nursing research. *Qualitative Report, 6*(2), 1–13. Retrieved from http://www.nova.edu/ssss/QR/QR6-2/zucker.html

CHAPTER 7

Qualitative Descriptive Projects

OBJECTIVES

At the end of this chapter, you will be able to:

- Explain the use of qualitative descriptive (QD) methods in doctor of nursing practice (DNP) projects.
- Compare and contrast qualitative and quantitative methods.
- Explain purposive sampling.
- Plan and conduct a focus group.

KEY CONCEPTS

- QD studies provide direct descriptions of a phenomenon.
- QD methods are based on naturalistic inquiry.
- Focus groups are typically used to collect data for a QD study.
- Focus group moderators need to be skilled communicators.

INTRODUCTION

Qualitative studies investigate experiences, social processes, meaning, perceptions, cultures, and context by entering a person's world and allowing the person's words to lead to greater understanding (Munhall, 2007). Descriptive studies, on the other hand, are typically associated with quantitative studies, but are basically summaries. Together these two types of studies combine to form the QD method, whose goal is a "comprehensive summary of events in the everyday terms of those events" (Sandelowski, 2000, p. 335), in other words, a description of events using the words and examples of the respondent. QD is the preferred method when an uncomplicated description is desired. Specific questions that provide undeviating descriptions of the phenomenon of interest guide the study. The more common approach is to view a QD study as exploratory. Questions are very broad, for example, "What are the factors that influence health policy in low-income countries?" or "What do patients think about electronic health records?" or "What strategies work best to sustain quality-improvement efforts?" Getting an answer might involve interviews, observation, and/or reviewing documents. Those engaging in a QD study "stay close to their data and to the surface of words and events" (Sandelowski, 2000, p. 337). In other words, interpretations of the results are of "low inference" with findings presented as a digest of the facts. Providing information that is of low inference means that you are only describing what you see or have been told. For example, if you describe the behavior of a chief nursing officer (CNO) as visionary, you are inferring that the CNO is imaginative, creative, and bold. This is an interpretation of the CNO's behavior, rather than a description. In a QD study, the behaviors of the CNO would be described as they occurred.

A QD inquiry is an effort to learn more about poorly understood phenomena. The inquiries are based on direct descriptions from (or observations of) the people who have experienced the phenomenon. Samples sizes are small. Data are most often derived from loosely structured interviews with study participants in either individual or group interviews. Data analysis is broad and generally does not follow a formal system such as constant comparison.

The primary aim of a QD study is to provide an accurate description of an event and the importance a subject applies to that event. There is minimal theorizing, as the QD researcher is interested in obtaining straight answers to questions (Sandelowski, 2000). For example, Carusone, Loeb, and Lohfeld (2006), in a study of what nursing home residents think about pneumonia care provided in a nursing home, interviewed only those residents deemed capable of remembering and discussing care provided for a recent case of pneumonia.

There are three types of QD study:

■ Definitional studies provide a greater understanding of a particular phenomenon. Definitional studies examine the nature of a phenomenon and its defining features. For example:
  What does it mean for patients with head and neck cancer to engage with a support group?

What are the experiences of students returning to school following a sports-related concussion?
■ Descriptive studies describe how a phenomenon appears.
For example:
How do Hispanic adults incorporate cultural food preferences into diabetes self-care?
How is a palliative care consult incorporated into the end-of-life care of those in a nursing home?
■ Critical/action studies provide a greater understanding about what is right or wrong with a phenomenon and ways it could be made better.
For example:
What concerns do faculty have about online testing?
What do nursing assistants perceive as risk for injury when using safe patient handling and mobility technology?

CHARACTERISTICS OF QD RESEARCH

A QD study differs from other qualitative methods in several ways. First, the aim of qualitative description is neither thick description (ethnography), theory development (grounded theory), nor interpretative meaning of an experience (phenomenology). Second, if an interview is conducted to collect data, the interview guide is more structured and questions are asked that relate specifically to the experience or event being investigated. Third, quality description is the least theoretical of the qualitative approaches. It is a way of gaining a beginning understanding of an informant's views on a specific topic (Neergaard, Olesen, Andersen, & Sondergaard, 2009). This may make the analytical process somewhat subjective, as descriptions will always depend on the researcher's perceptions and preferences (Sandelowski, 2000). Reflexivity is an important consideration used to avoid this bias. Reflexivity involves reflecting upon the ways in which one's own values, experiences, interests, and beliefs can bias the research (Box 7.1). Finally, quality description is less time- consuming than other qualitative methods.

The QD method is not bound by theoretical assumptions as other qualitative methodologies are, such as grounded theory in sociology, phenomenology in philosophy, or ethnography in anthropology. A QD study is based in naturalistic inquiry, the study of something in its own unique environment. According to Erlander, Harris, Skipper, and Allen (1993), the problem statement in a naturalistic inquiry does not have to be a question or even an objective; rather, it is an "expression of a

BOX 7.1

REFLEXIVITY IN QUALITATIVE DESCRIPTIVE STUDIES

Reflexivity involves reflecting upon the ways in which your own values, experiences, interests, and beliefs can bias the research. To engage in reflection and decrease bias, the QD researcher must:

1. Carefully consider the interview conducted and how much influence the researcher may have had on the conversations. The researcher must be able to ensure that personal perceptions and assumptions did not sway the findings.
2. Get the help of an assistant to observe the researcher during focus group interviews, to limit bias and researcher influence.
3. Conduct an audit with the assistant to corroborate how she or he arrived at the findings (to increase the validity of findings).

QD, qualitative description.

dilemma or a situation that needs to be addressed for the purposes of understanding" (p. 49). The focus is about how people understand or think about events or experiences with consideration as to how and why during the interview. The value of this approach is its ability to raise questions and provide a foundation for construction of hypotheses.

CONDUCTING A QD STUDY

Planning a QD study involves attention to sampling, data collection, and data analysis.

Sampling

A qualitative study is not concerned with determining the significance of findings or confidence intervals. Instead, qualitative research typically tries to sample the population. Nor is it concerned with power analysis or sample size. Generalizability of results is replaced with a focus on applicability of findings. Because the primary aim of a QD study is a straightforward representation of an event or experience, a purposive sample is generally used. Purposive sampling seeks to find subjects who have some specific knowledge or expertise relevant to the topic; in other words they are rich in the information needed for the study. There are many approaches to purposive sampling; however, maximum variation sampling (MVS), a type of purposive sampling, allows for the greatest diversity among subjects. MVS does not seek representativeness through equal probabilities; rather, this type of sampling seeks to include those with a wide range of extremes in opinions or experiences, which allows for broader understanding of the topic of interest. The assumption is that if you deliberately try to interview a very diverse selection of people, their aggregate answers can be close to the whole population and can be as representative as a random sample (List, 2004). When using MVS, all the extremes in the population should be represented. For example, on a nursing unit for a study on how well a new protocol on bedside reporting is working, it is beneficial to conduct interviews with the nurse or nurses:

- With the most years of experience
- With the least years of experience
- Who have indicated that bedside reporting is working well
- Who have never given bedside reporting
- Who have expressed a dislike for bedside reporting
- Who have little to say about bedside reporting

Data Collection

Data collection in QD studies is directed toward discovering the who, what, and where of events or experiences. Data-collection methods typically involve the use of focus groups, document review, or observation of a specific event (Table 7.1). Focus groups are the most common data-collection tool used.

FOCUS GROUPS

Focus groups are discussions around a predetermined set of questions. Focus group questions are related to a specific topic or event. Focus group sessions should be audiotaped. The researcher (called a *moderator*) should have an assistant available to be sure that the recording device works properly and to assist in taking field notes and attend to the logistics of the focus group (e.g., room temperature, refreshments). The role of the moderator is to keep the conversation going and to reduce any unrelated conversation. The moderator should be friendly and greet each person in the focus group. One of the important functions of the moderator is to ensure that no one member of the group dominates and that all group members have the opportunity to contribute

TABLE 7.1

METHODS OF DATA COLLECTION

Method	Description	Advantages	Limitations
Focus group interview	Focus groups are interviews of a group of containing 6–10 participants. Each focus group session should last 1–2 hours.	Findings emerge from a group with a special interest or expertise in the topic. Findings can provide a foundation for further study or instrument development.	Subjects are not equally articulate. Transcripts may be extensive and difficult to analyze. The small group size limits generalizability.
Observation	Observation is the researcher's attempt to note and record all behaviors of interest to an investigation.	Observations are recorded as they occur so that there is no loss of information. Observation overcomes the discrepancy between what people say they do and what they actually do.	The researcher may be seen as intrusive. Only current observations or behaviors can be identified. Sampled time frames (e.g., 3 minutes or 1 hour) may not correspond to real-life events.
Document review	A review of recorded information that is relevant to the investigation, such as reports, memos, meeting minutes, etc.	Can confirm information gathered during interview or observation.	May not be accessible. Documents may be incomplete or poorly written.

to the session. A moderator needs to remain neutral; one who appears to be an expert on the subject will close important avenues of discussion. The moderator must have the ability to use participants' words and statements to introduce new topics and refer to what participants have said as a basis for moving to the next topic or question. See Box 7.2 for

BOX 7.2

MODERATOR SKILLS

Ability to communicate clearly
Ability to listen, not talk
Ability to avoid expressing personal views
Ability to maintain a low level of involvement
Ability to listen
Ability to remember what was discussed

other necessary skills of a moderator. Some materials needed for a focus group session are:

- Notepads and pencils
- Recording device
- Flip chart or easel paper
- Focus group questions
- List of participants
- Markers
- Masking tape
- Name tags
- Refreshments
- Watch

The focus group should consist of six to 10 participants. Fewer than six participants tends to limit the conversation, and a group larger than 10 makes it difficult for the researcher to keep the discussion on track and to record nonverbal communication. A focus group should last between 1 and 2 hours, which is enough time for five to 10 questions (see Box 7.3 for sample focus group questions). The actual amount of time needed depends upon the sample. Children, for example, may only be able to participate for no more than an hour. Questions should include some introductory or icebreaker questions, which are asked first (see Box 7.4 for examples of icebreakers). The best focus group questions are open ended, and the researcher will have some prompts ready to keep the conversation moving, which means that the facilitator needs to be very familiar with the questions

BOX 7.3

SAMPLE FOCUS GROUP QUESTIONS

Study question: What do school-aged children think about obesity?
Time frame: 1 hour

Focus Group Question 1
Let's begin by going around the room one at a time. Please start by telling us your name and your favorite activities.

Focus Group Question 2
What does the word *obesity* mean to you?
Possible prompts:

■ What does an obese person look like?

Focus Group Question 3
How do you think people become obese or _____ (insert a word the children used to describe obesity?
Possible prompts:

■ Can you give me an example?

Focus Group Question 4
Do you know anyone who is obese?
Possible prompts:

■ (If so,) What caused this to happen?

Focus Group Question 5
How do you think it feels to be obese?
Possible prompts:

■ Can you tell me more about that?

Focus Group Question 6
Would anyone like to share anything else?

to be asked. Prompts can be detail oriented, such as, "When did this event happen to you?"; elaborative, such as, "Tell me more about that"; or clarifying, such as, "I'm not sure I understand what you mean by *onboarding* of new nurses. Can you explain?"

Questions should move from the general, "What do you think about . . .?" to the specific, "What can be done about that?" The questions should match the purpose of the study. The setting in which the focus group takes place should be accessible, encourage conversation, and

BOX 7.4

ICEBREAKERS

Who Knew?
Go around the room and ask everyone to tell the group something about themselves that no one in the room knows.

Sentence Completion
These can be put on a flip chart or white board. Ask participants to complete the following sentences:
"If I could throw caution to the wind, I would . . ."
"If I could be any person, alive or dead, it would be . . ."
"I laugh when . . ."
"I cry when . . ."

Who Am I?
Go around the group and ask each person to write his or her name on a label along with a personal characteristic that starts with the same letter as his or her name, for example, Shy Sally or Dynamic Dennis.

comfortably seat 10 to 12 people who can easily view each other. When the last question has been asked, the moderator should begin to end the focus group session by summarizing the discussion and asking participants whether they wish to share anything else. This is also the time for the moderator to clarify anything that was unclear and to verify the accuracy of the information discussed. The analysis process should begin immediately following the focus group session with a written summary of the session. The moderator and assistant should share perceptions of the process and compare field notes. The tapes should be transcribed as soon after the focus group discussion as possible.

DOCUMENT REVIEW
Documents refers to any preserved recording. They can provide confirmation of information obtained from interviews and observations. A document review is the appraisal of textual information. Textual information can include letters, newspaper articles, reports, memos, meeting minutes, and so on. For example, in a study of nurse retention, exit interviews of nurses who left the organization would be considered a document. In some cases, a segmental review is necessary, as all of the document may not be relevant to the study. Information

retrieved from documents needs to relate to the study purpose. This is called the *recording unit*. Documents that are vague or incomplete may need to be discarded due to serious doubts about the quality of the document.

OBSERVATION

Observation is the act of watching. For example, if you want to investigate what goes on in the nurses' lounge, you can sit in the lounge for a specified length of time and record observations. You can see and hear what nurses are concerned about. Observation is a good source of information for studies involving infants or young children, the mentally ill, or incapacitated persons, particularly when the variables of interest are physical or behavioral. Observation is also an important method for determining reactions to new treatments or compliance with new protocols. For example, observing the behavior of a patient for 2 hours after ingestion of a new drug will allow the researcher to determine whether any unexpected reactions occurred as a result of the drug. As QD study is exploratory, extended periods of observation may be necessary, and the observer needs to be sure that nothing is missed during the observation. Questions to ask when constructing an observation include:

- How long should the observation last?
- How often should each participant be observed?
- When should the observation be done?
- How should observations be recorded?

Data Analysis

Content analysis is used for QD studies to construct codes and themes. Content analysis is used to determine the frequency of words in transcriptions, documents, or observations. Coding is the first step in content analysis and provides its foundation. An original quote is a code. Several similar codes constitute a theme or a single assertion about a topic that shows the relationship to the codes. This method provides a means of measuring the frequency and order of words, phrases, or sentences within a specific context (Gray, Grove, & Sutherland, 2012; Figure 7.1).

To perform a content analysis, the verbatim transcriptions of interviews, the recording units of the document review, and the observations made, are coded, line by line. There are computer software programs that will code data (e.g., NIVO), but some qualitative researchers will code their own data using colored highlighters or sticky notes. According

18 The pain was so excruciating that I thought my head would explode. I could not

19 think or move or respond in any way. The pain was tremendous. It was unforgettable.

20 I agree, I felt the same way when I had a stroke. The pain was one of the single most terrifying

21 experiences of my life. I thought the world was ending as I knew it. Sometimes, even now, when

22 I think back to that day, I can still feel the pain, even though people have told me I would forget

23 how bad it was. I have not forgotten.

Word count

Pain 5 = 4

Forget/unforgettable/not forgotten 5 = 3

Theme: Unforgettable pain

FIGURE 7.1 Code passage from a study on perceptions of pain.

to Krippendorff (2004), six questions must be addressed in every content analysis:

1. Which data are analyzed?
2. How are they defined?
3. What is the population from which they are drawn?
4. What is the context relative to which the data are analyzed?
5. What are the boundaries of the analysis?
6. What is the target of the inferences?

As themes are developed, the researcher assigns a working definition to each code. That way, in going through the transcripts or other recorded results, the definition is continually challenged. New codes may have to be developed as they do not fit into the definition of existing ones. This is a circular method of analysis as the researchers go round and round among codes, themes, and definitions. This process is ongoing until saturation is reached, a state when no new codes or categories emerge and coding anything else would only produce repetition of themes.

To enhance the validity of qualitative findings, the following strategies should be considered:

1. Triangulation, which is the cross-checking of information from different dimensions, can be used. For example, at the end of a focus group session, the moderator can summarize the discussion

and ask the participants whether the summary captured the essential elements of the session. The moderator and the focus group assistant can also compare field notes recorded during the session.

2. Longer or multiple observations that can provide a more accurate picture of the phenomenon of interest than just a short or single observation should be encouraged.
3. Use member checking, the review of findings with a subgroup of those who were interviewed, to verify accuracy.
4. Keep an audit trail, a detailed and accurate record of everything the researcher does throughout the study.

WRITING THE QUALITATIVE RESEARCH REPORT

The qualitative research report follows the traditional standards used for writing research reports: abstract, introduction, aims of the study, review of the literature, sample, data-collection methods, data-analysis methods, findings, discussion, and conclusions. However, as it is a subjective method of research, dealing primarily with words and descriptions, it is necessary to communicate as clearly as possible what was done; the details of the design; how data were collected, transcribed, and categorized; and how final themes or descriptions were generated. This allows the reader to judge the credibility of the findings. The main focus should be on the data. Participants should be generously quoted to illustrate a category.

CONCLUSIONS

QD projects consist of a broad inquiry that uses unstructured data-collection methods, such as focus groups, observations, or documents. A QD design is used when an uncomplicated description is desired that focuses on the details of the what, where, when, and why of an event or experience. Interpretation of these descriptions is not an aspect of this type of project.

■ QUESTIONS FOR DISCUSSION

1. Choose a public place to sit in for an hour, for example, the library, a train station, a shopping mall, or a coffee shop. Observe the people you see. Write a description of what you see. Do not

try to interpret what you think those you observed were doing; just describe what you see using everyday language.

2. Describe a clinical problem that would lend itself to greater understanding using a QD approach.

■ REFLECTIVE EXERCISES

1. Reflect on the following list of potential QD studies. Select one and write a research question and list of focus group interview questions for the study.
   a. An evaluation of a nurse-managed clinic
   b. The role of psychiatric nurse practitioners in group sessions
   c. The leadership style of CNOs
   d. The experience of returning to work after head and neck surgery for cancer
2. Examine the biographical data of 10 nursing faculty members at any university. What are the common themes you see in these data?

EXAMPLE OF A QD PROJECT

Nursing Students' Perceptions of a Collaborative Clinical Placement Model: A QD Study
Collaborative placement models, grounded in a tripartite relationship among students, university staff, and clinical partners and designed to foster students' sense of belonging, have recently been implemented to address many of the challenges associated with clinical placements. In this study a QD design was undertaken with the aim of exploring 14 third-year nursing students' perceptions of a collaborative clinical placement model. Students participated in audio-recorded focus groups following their final clinical placement. Thematic analysis of the interview data resulted in identification of six main themes: convenience and camaraderie, familiarity and confidence, welcomed and wanted, belongingness and support, employment, and the need for broader clinical experiences. The clinical collaborative model fostered a sense of familiarity for many of the participants and this led to belongingness, acceptance, confidence, and meaningful learning experiences.

Reference
van der Riet, P., Levett-Jones, T., & Courtney-Pratt, H. (2018). Nursing students' perceptions of a collaborative clinical placement model: A qualitative descriptive study. *Nurse Education in Practice, 30*, 42–47. doi:10.1016/j.nepr.2018.02.007

■ SUGGESTED READINGS

Burnard, P. (2004). Writing a qualitative research report. *Accident and Emergency Nursing, 12,* 176–181. doi:10.1016/j.aaen.2003.11.006

Hanson, S. E., MacLeod, M. L., & Schiller, C. J. (2018). "It's complicated": Staff nurse perceptions of their influence on nursing students' learning. A qualitative descriptive study. *Nurse Education Today, 63,* 76–80. doi:10.1016/j.nedt.2018.01.017

Mauthner, N. S., & Doucet, A. (2011). Reflexive accounts and accounts of reflexivity in qualitative data analysis. *Sociology, 37*(3), 413–431. doi:10.1177/00380385030373002

Sandelowski, M. (2000). Whatever happened to qualitative descriptive. *Nursing in Research and Health, 23,* 334–340. doi:10.1002/1098-240X(200008)23:43.0.CO;2-G

■ REFERENCES

Carusone, S. C., Loeb, M., & Lohfeld, L. (2006). Pneumonia care and the nursing home: A qualitative descriptive study of resident and family member perspectives. *BMC Geriatrics, 6,* 2.

Erlander, D., Harris, E., Skipper, B., & Allen, S. (1993). *Doing naturalistic inquiry: A guide to methods.* Thousand Oaks, CA: Sage.

Gray, J., Grove, S., & Sutherland, S. (2017). *Burns and Grove's the practice of nursing research.* (8th ed.). Philadelphia, PA: Saunders.

Krippendorff, K. (2004). *Content analysis: An introduction to its methodology* (2nd ed.). Thousand Oaks, CA: Sage.

List, D. (2004). *Maximum variation sampling for surveys and consensus groups.* Adelaide, Australia: Audience Dialogue. Retrieved from www.audiencedialogue.org/maxvar.html

Munhall, P. (2007). *The landscape of qualitative research.* Sudbury, MA: Jones & Bartlett.

Neergaard, M. A., Olesen, F., Andersen, R. S., & Sondergaard, J. (2009). Qualitative description—The poor cousin of health research? *BMC Medical Research Methodology, 9,* 52.

Sandelowski, M. (2000). Whatever happened to qualitative descriptive. *Nursing in Research and Health, 23,* 334–340. doi:10.1002/1098-240X(200008)23:43.0.CO;2-G

CHAPTER 8

Clinical Interventional Studies

■ OBJECTIVES

At the end of this chapter, you will be able to:

- Identify the steps in a clinical interventional study.
- Compare and contrast preexperimental designs, quasi-experimental designs, and true experimental designs.
- Understand the basic statistical principles, concepts, and methods for analysis of clinical interventional data.
- Design strategies to ensure fidelity of the intervention.

■ KEY CONCEPTS

There are three basic interventional designs:

- Preexperimental design
- Quasi-experimental design
- True experimental design

Interventional research studies involve manipulation of the independent variable (IV).

Interventional studies build knowledge about what works and does not work given specific conditions and subject characteristics.

A clinical intervention is any deliberate physical, educational, or verbal action directed toward accomplishing a particular goal.

Demonstrating the fidelity of an intervention is a key methodological requirement of any good interventional study.

INTRODUCTION

An interventional study is a type of clinical study in which participants (or subjects) are assigned to groups that receive one or more intervention or treatment (or no intervention) so that the effects of the intervention can be evaluated. Interventional studies use the scientific method to build knowledge. Building clinical knowledge in nursing implies having an understanding of the person: as an individual or as a member of a family. The focus of a clinical interventional study can also be a community or a group or a program. An intervention is a single act, a series of actions at either one point in time or over a period of time, or collaborative actions with other professionals (Burns & Grove, 2009). Forbes (2009) defines a *clinical intervention* as an explicit act, treatment, or technology (physical, psychological, or social) focused on a specific patient (or healthcare) problem or need. Any of the following can be an intervention: taking a blood pressure (a single act) reading, caring for a severely injured patient in the ED (a series of actions at one point in time), implementing a protocol to decrease urinary tract infections (a series of actions over time), or installing an electronic health record (EHR) system (collaborating with other professionals).

Nursing interventions must be completely described and fit within a theoretical or conceptual framework. (See Box 8.1 for a list of commonly used terms.) Thus, clinical interventional research is guided by theory. Theory, according to Fleury and Sidani (2012), "provides an understanding of the problem the intervention targets, the nature of the intervention, and the mechanisms underlying anticipated improvement in outcomes" (p. 11). Framing interventions with a theory acknowledges the importance of how the concepts fit together to influence outcomes. "Without a theory serving as (a) guide, choosing which constructs to investigate and manipulate would be like going on a wild goose chase" (Melnyk, Morrison-Beedy, & Moore, 2012, p. 49).

The choice of the right theory to use to frame a clinical interventional study begins with identifying the problem, goal, or aspect of practice to be investigated, not selecting the theory because it is familiar or popular. Different theories are best suited to different targets, such as individuals, groups, and organizations (National Institutes of Health [NIH], 2013). For example, when implementing a smoking-cessation program, the transtheoretical model may be useful. When installing a new EHR system throughout a facility, Rogers's diffusion of innovation theory may be the best to use. Organizational change theory may work well when trying to change practice patterns (NIH, 2013). See Table 8.1 for examples of theories used in clinical interventional studies.

BOX 8.1

GLOSSARY OF COMMON TERMS USED IN INTERVENTIONAL STUDIES

Adverse event
An unfavorable change in the health of a participant, including abnormal laboratory findings, that occurs during a clinical study or within a certain amount of time after the study has ended.

Age or age group
A type of eligibility criteria that indicates the age a person must be to participate in a study. This may be indicated by a specific age or the following age groups.

■ Child (birth–17)
■ Adult (18–64)
■ Older adult (65+)

Allocation
A method used to assign participants to an arm of a clinical study. The types of allocation are randomized and nonrandomized allocation.

Arm
A group or subgroup of participants in a clinical trial that receives a specific intervention/treatment, or no intervention, according to the protocol.

Baseline characteristics
These are data collected on all participants at the beginning of a clinical study and for each arm or comparison group. These data include demographics, such as age, gender, race, and ethnicity, and study-specific measures (e.g., systolic blood pressure, prior antidepressant treatment).

Cross-over
A type of interventional model describing a clinical trial in which groups of participants receive two or more interventions in a specific order. For example, a two-by-two cross-over assignment involves two groups of participants. One group receives Intervention A first, followed by Intervention B. The other group receives Intervention B first, followed by Intervention A. Participants "cross over" to the other intervention. They all receive the same interventions, but in a different order.

Eligibility criteria
These refer to the key requirements that people must meet or the characteristics they must have to be in the study. Eligibility criteria consist of both inclusion criteria (which are required for a person to participate in the study) and exclusion criteria (which prevent a person from participating).

Experimental arm
This refers to the group of participants that receives the intervention/treatment that is the focus of the clinical trial.

Group/cohort
A set or subset of participants in an observational study who are assessed for biomedical or health outcomes.

(continued)

BOX 8.1 *(CONTINUED)*

Intervention design/model
　　This is the general design of the strategy for assigning interventions to participants. The types of intervention models include single group assignment, parallel assignment, cross-over assignment, and factorial assignment.

Intervention/treatment
　　A process or action that is the focus of a clinical study. Interventions can be invasive or noninvasive, such as with use of medical devices, procedures, vaccines, education, or modifying diet and exercise.

No intervention arms
　　An arm type in which a group of participants do not receive any intervention/treatment during the clinical trial.

Observational study
　　A type of study in which participants are identified as belonging to study groups and are assessed for health outcomes. Participants may receive diagnostic, therapeutic, or other types of interventions, but the investigator does not assign participants to a specific intervention/treatment.

Outcome measure
　　A planned measurement described in the protocol used to determine the effect of an intervention/treatment on participants. For observational studies, a measurement or observation that is used to describe patterns of diseases or traits or associations with exposures, risk factors, or treatment. The types of outcome measures include primary outcome measure and secondary outcome measure.

Primary outcome measure
　　The planned outcome measure that is the most important for evaluating the effect of an intervention/treatment. Most clinical studies have one primary outcome measure.

Primary purpose
　　This is the main reason for the clinical trial. The types of primary purpose are treatment, prevention, diagnostic, supportive care, screening, health services research, basic science, and other.

Protocol
　　This refers to the written description of a clinical study. It includes the study's objectives, design, and methods. It may also include relevant scientific background and statistical information.

Randomized allocation
　　A type of allocation strategy in which participants are assigned to the arms of a clinical trial by chance.

Secondary outcome measure
　　A planned outcome measure that is not as important as the primary outcome measure for evaluating the effect of an intervention, but is still of interest. Most clinical studies have more than one secondary outcome measure.

Serious adverse event
　　An adverse event that results in death, is life-threatening, requires inpatient hospitalization or extends a current hospital stay, results in an ongoing or significant incapacity or interferes substantially with normal life functions, or causes a congenital anomaly or birth defect.

TABLE 8.1

EXAMPLES OF INTERVENTIONAL STUDIES USING A THEORETICAL FRAMEWORK

Reference	Intervention	Theory Used
Ibrahim, K., May, C. R., Patel, H. P., Baxter, M., Sayer, A. A., & Roberts, H. C. (2018). Implementation of grip strength measurement in medicine for older people wards as part of routine admission assessment: identifying facilitators and barriers using a theory-led intervention. *BMC Geriatrics, 18*(1), 79. doi:10.1186/s12877-018-0768-5	Training program	Normalization theory
Zhou, Y., Liao, J., Feng, F., Ji, M., Zhao, C., & Wang, X. (2018). Effects of a nurse-led phone follow-up education program based on the self-efficacy among patients with cardiovascular disease. *Journal of Cardiovascular Nursing, 33*(1), E15–E23. doi:10.1097/JCN.0000000000000414	Nurse-led follow-up telephone program	Self-efficacy
Meraviglia, M., Stuifbergen, A., Parsons, D., & Morgans, S. (2013). Health promotion for cancer survivors: Adaptation and implementation of an intervention. *Holistic Nursing Practice, 27*(3), 140–147. doi:10.1097/HNP.0b013e31828a0988	The three-component intervention included (a) development of one-on-one participant-provider support relationships, (b) attendance at six weekly classes, and (c) follow-up support for 2 months to encourage use of health-promoting behaviors	Health promotion with chronic conditions

(continued)

TABLE 8.1 (CONTINUED)

EXAMPLES OF INTERVENTIONAL STUDIES USING A THEORETICAL FRAMEWORK

Reference	Intervention	Theory Used
Navidian, A., & Bahari, F. (2013). The impact of mixed, hope and forgiveness-focused marital counselling on interpersonal cognitive distortions of couples filing for divorce. *Journal of Psychiatric and Mental Health Nursing, 21*, 658–666. doi:10.1111/jpm.12058	Counseling sessions	An integrated model of hope
Weatherspoon, D., & Wyatt, T. (2012). Testing computer-based simulation to enhance clinical judgment skills in senior nursing students. *Nursing Clinics of North America, 47*(4), 481–491. doi:10.1016/j.cnur.2012.07.002	Simulation	Kolb's experiential learning theory
Hoffman, A. J., Brintnall, R. A., Brown, J. K., Eye, A. V., Jones, L. W., Alderink, G., . . . Vanotteren, G. M. (2013). Too sick not to exercise: Using a 6-week, home-based exercise intervention for cancer-related fatigue self-management for postsurgical non-small cell lung cancer patients. *Cancer Nursing, 36*(3), 175–188. doi:10.1097/NCC.0b013e31826c7763	Low-intensity walking and balance exercises in a virtual reality environment with the Nintendo Wii Fit Plus	Symptom self-management
Paradis, V., Cossette, S., Smith, N., Heppell, S., & Guertin, M. C. (2010). The efficacy of a motivational nursing intervention based on the stages of change on self-care in heart failure patients. *Journal of Cardiovascular Nursing, 25*(2), 130–141. doi:10.1097/JCN.0b013e3181c52497	Motivational interviewing	Heart failure self-care

The relevance or significance of a theory to the target population and intervention needs to be considered. When determining the relevance of a theory to an interventional study, an evaluation of the theory's underlying assumptions, empirical support for the theory's propositions, concept definitions, and construct validity are essential.

DESIGNING INTERVENTIONAL STUDIES

A study design is a blueprint. Good study designs (a) answer the research question asked, (b) control for confounding variables, and (c) have a large enough sample to determine statistical significance (Melynk & Cole, 2011). There are three types of interventional research designs (Table 8.2): preexperimental designs, quasi-experimental designs, and experimental designs. Before any interventional study can begin, however, informed consent is necessary (Box 8.2).

Preexperiments are inexpensive and the simplest form of research. This preexperiment is used to determine whether a particular area of study is worthy of further investigation. Although preexperimental designs follow basic experimental steps, they do not have a control group. A disadvantage of preexperimental designs is that they are subject to numerous threats to validity, making it difficult to eliminate the possibility of competing explanations. Examples include the following:

THE ONE-SHOT CASE STUDY
In this type of study, subjects are presented with a treatment, such as the effect of simulation on knowledge attainment. The aim is to determine whether the treatment (simulation) had any effect on the outcome (knowledge); however, there is no comparison group and no baseline testing. Without a comparison group, it is impossible to determine whether the outcome (knowledge attainment) is any higher than it would have been without the treatment.

ONE GROUP PRETEST–POSTTEST STUDY
In this type of study, pretest data are collected. For example, in the study of simulation on knowledge attainment, an exam could be given prior to the simulation and then again after the simulation, which can indicate a change in knowledge levels. It is still not possible, however, to be able to know whether the change is as a result of the treatment (simulation).

TABLE 8.2

TYPES OF RESEARCH DESIGNS

Design	Focus	Elements	Learn More
Preexperimental	Exploration	Little is known about the topic under investigation. In preexperimental designs, either a single group of participants or multiple groups are observed after some intervention or treatment presumed to cause change. Although they do follow some basic steps used in experiments, preexperimental designs fail to include either a pretest or a control or comparison group, or both; in addition, no randomization procedures are used to control for extraneous variables. Thus, they are considered *pre*, indicating they are preparatory or prerequisite to true experimental designs. Preexperimental designs represent the simplest form of research designs. Together with quasi-experimental designs and true experimental (also called *randomized experimental*) designs, they comprise the three basic categories of designs used with an intervention.	Wyatt, T., & Hauenstein, E. (2008). Pilot: An online asthma intervention for school aged children. *Journal of School Nursing, 24*(3), 145–150. doi:10.1177/1059840522334455 Design: One group pretest–posttest

| Quasi-experimental | Description | Depicts a topic through data collected to answer a research question or test a hypothesis. Lacks randomization. | Muntlin, A., Carlsso, M., Safwenberg, U., & Gunningberg, L. (2011). Outcomes of a nurse-initiated intravenous analgesic protocol for abdominal pain in an emergency department: A quasi-experimental study. *International Journal of Nursing Studies, 48*(1), 13–23. doi:10.1016/j.ijnurstu.2010.06.003 |
| Experimental | Explanation | Independent variables are used to assign subjects to interventional and comparison groups. At least one variable is manipulated to test the effect on the outcome of interest. | Mathey, M., Vanneste, V., Graaf, C., deGroot, L., & van Staeren, W. (2001). Health of improved meal ambiance in a Dutch nursing home: A 1-year intervention study. *Preventive Medicine, 32*(5), 416–423. doi:10.1006/pmed.2001.0816 |

BOX 8.2

ELEMENTS OF AN INFORMED CONSENT

Title of the study
Purpose of the study
Name of the researchers involved in the study
Affiliation of researchers
Procedures
Requirements of the subject
How information will be used
Potential benefit
Potential harm (risk of participating)
Statement on ability to withdraw without consequence
Signature of subject and witness
Date

STATIC-GROUP COMPARISON

This design compares the outcomes of two naturally occurring groups, such as two nursing units or two classrooms. The groups remain intact. One group receives the experimental treatment, and the other does not. Both groups are then measured. The researcher then compares the two sets of measurements to see whether there is a difference. This design attempts to make up for the lack of a control group; however, lack of a pretest does not allow the researcher to determine wheher the intervention made any difference.

Quasi-experimental designs have both an experimental and a comparison group; however, subjects are assigned, rather than randomized, to groups. Quasi-experimental studies include:

PRETEST–POSTTEST NONEQUIVALENT GROUP

In this design, there is both a control group and an experimental group. This might be the method of choice used for the simulation study. Students could be asked to participate in a one-semester simulation experience, in which the simulation would take the place of some clinical hours, followed by measurement of knowledge. Knowledge would be measured prior to the simulation and again after the program ended. Those students who participated in the simulation would be the treatment group; those who did not would be the control group.

TIME SERIES DESIGNS

Time series designs refer to the pretesting and posttesting of one group of subjects at different intervals. The purpose is to determine the long-term effect of the intervention; therefore, the number of pre- and posttests can vary from one each to many. In the simulation study, for example, knowledge could be measured immediately after the intervention, at 3 months, 6 months, and 1 year to determine whether the knowledge was sustained. When there is an interruption between tests to assess the strength of the intervention over an extended time period, the posttest is referred to as *follow-up* and the design is called an *interrupted time series*.

Experimental design employs both an intervention group and a control group as well as a means to measure the change that occurs in both groups. There is an attempt to control for confounding variables, or at least consider their impact on the outcome, while attempting to determine whether the treatment is what caused the change. The true experiment is often thought of as the only research method that can adequately measure cause and effect. Examples of this type of design include:

POSTTEST EQUIVALENT GROUPS STUDY

In this study design, there is both an experimental and a control group. Group assignment is done randomly. Posttests are given to each subject after the intervention to determine whether a difference between the two groups exists. There is no pretest measure.

PRETEST–POSTTEST EQUIVALENT GROUPS STUDY

This method is the most effective in demonstrating cause and effect, but it is also the most difficult, most time-consuming, and most costly to perform. The pretest–posttest equivalent groups design provides for both a control group and an experimental group and adds a pretest. To apply this design to the simulation study, students would be selected randomly and then placed in either the intervention group or control group. The intervention (simulation) would be applied to one group and a control (usual method of teaching) would be applied to the other. It is important that the two groups be treated in a similar manner.

Prior to using any of these designs, the intervention or experiment must be planned and tested to the extent possible. Planning involves a determination regarding who will be involved in the intervention, including the need for any stakeholders (e.g., patients), whereas testing may require practice sessions or a pilot test. An intervention (also called a *treatment*) can be any of the following (Burns & Grove, 2009):

■ A strategy
■ A technique
■ A program
■ Training materials
■ Methods of motivation
■ Policy implementation

The way in which the intervention is to be administered should be guided by an intervention protocol. The protocol can be supplemented by an intervention manual and fact sheets. The manual should include a description of the topic, including its theoretical foundation and a reference list. The activities to be conducted as a part of the intervention, any needed equipment, and the mode of delivery should be clearly described in the protocol. Any necessary handouts should also be included with a timeline as to when they should be distributed. The manual can contain standards for the intervention in terms of dose (i.e., the frequency and duration of the intervention). Depending upon the intervention, it may be necessary to provide a verbatim script. Strategies for reinforcing key ideas, troubleshooting, and actions for dealing with unhappy participants can also be included. The manual should also contain a list of names and contact information if any questions or concerns arise during the course of the intervention. The advantage of developing and using a manual is the greater consistency and precision with which the intervention will be delivered, which enhances internal validity (Santacroce, Mararelli, & Grey, 2004). The manual should also contain directions and forms for recording the number, frequency, and duration of all subject contacts as well as any deviations from the protocol (Fleury & Sidani, 2012).

Those who are administering the intervention should be formally trained and supervised prior to the start of the study. According to Santacroce, Macarelli, and Grey (2004), "the purpose of training and supervision is to mold, refine, and expand the skills of professionals who have experience with the study population or type of intervention. Training and supervision are achieved through manual review, didactic seminars, and experience" (p. 65). Attention to the training of those who are implementing the intervention is necessary to ensure that the intervention is conducted as planned, known as *fidelity*. An intervention can be said to satisfy fidelity requirements if it can be shown that each of its components is delivered in a comparable manner to all participants and is true to the theory guiding the intervention and the research aims. Demonstrating the fidelity of an intervention is a key methodological requirement of any good intervention study (Dumas, Lynch, Laughlin, Smith, & Prinz, 2001).

VARIABLES AND HYPOTHESES

Every interventional study has at least two types of variables: independent and dependent. The IV can be manipulated. An IV causes a dependent variable (DV) to react. An example of an IV is noise level. Noise levels can be kept very low (a library whisper) or very high (a jackhammer), and the level of noise can be measured in decibels. Response to noise levels would be the DV, as the way someone would react to a certain level of noise can be related to the type and/or volume of the noise. The results of the study would depend on how the test subjects reacted to the noise. Measurements could include heart rate, respiratory rate, anxiety or anger level, or galvanic skin response. Any variable that can influence the outcome of a study but is not part of the study is called a *confounding variable*. For example, a loud clap of thunder that occurs during the noise-level study could interfere with results, as its level of noise cannot be controlled.

The hypothesis is directly related to the guiding theory used in the study, but contains operationally defined variables in measurable form. A hypothesis is a single sentence that expresses the possible relationship between variables. The null hypothesis (H_0) is what is tested by statistics. Because the null is being tested, it is believed that if the null hypothesis is not true, then some alternative to the null must be true. The alternative hypothesis (H_1) is also called the *research hypothesis* because it is really the aim of the investigation. To conclude that there is no difference between the two groups' means is an acceptance of the null hypothesis. However, if statistical testing shows that the null hypothesis is not true, then it is rejected, and the alternative hypothesis is accepted, that is, there is a difference between the group means. For example:

H_0: Noise at 120 decibels (amplified rock music) will have no effect on heart rate.

H_1: Noise at 120 decibels (amplified rock music) will increase heart rate.

VALIDITY OF INTERVENTIONAL STUDIES

A valid study represents what it was intended to represent. There are two types of validity: (1) internal validity and (2) external validity. *Internal validity* refers to the ability to determine whether a causal relationship exists between one or more IVs and one or more DVs. In other words, did the treatment really affect the outcome, either positively or negatively? There are eight major threats to internal validity, including:

History. *History* refers to any event outside of the research study that can change or affect a subject's performance. This threat can be controlled by randomization.

Maturation. *Maturation* refers to the usual physiological or psychological changes that take place as a result of aging. It can be controlled by subject matching so that all subjects mature equally. Randomization also helps to control this threat.

Testing. *Testing* refers to the use of the same test before and after the intervention. The chances that subjects will perform better the second time are a concern. Use of a control group can help with this threat.

Statistical Regression. *Statistical regression*, or *regression to the mean*, refers to the tendency for subjects who score very high or very low to score more toward the mean on subsequent testing. This can be addressed by dropping the outliers from analysis, that is, those who score very low or very high.

Instrumentation. This threat refers to a change in the measurement tool used in a study. Changes in scores may be related to the difference in tools rather than the IV. For instance, if a pretest is different than a posttest, the change in scores may be a result of the second test being easier or harder. This threat can be addressed by ensuring that alternative forms of testing are reliable and equivocal.

Selection. *Selection* refers to the manner in which subjects are selected to participate in a study and the manner in which they are assigned to groups. This threat can be addressed by randomizing subjects to study groups.

Experimenter Bias. This bias can affect results that skew the study in the direction wanted. It can be controlled through blinding.

Mortality. Mortality, or subject dropout, is always a concern and can be controlled by subject matching.

External validity refers to the generalizability of a study. In other words, can we be sure that the results of our study population represent the entire population? There are four major threats to external validity:

Demand Characteristics. Demand characteristics involve inadvertently letting the subjects know the hypotheses under study. When asked a series of questions about work environments and burnout, for example, subjects may be cued to the hypothesis. When subjects become wise to anticipated results (a placebo effect), they may exhibit behaviors that they believe are expected of them. This threat can be controlled by blinding and the use of control groups.

Hawthorne Effects. The act of watching a performance can cause a change in that performance, as those being watched may want to perform at a higher level. This can be controlled by use of a control group.

Order Effects. *Order effects* refer to the order in which interventions are administered. According to Cohen (1995, para 1),

> performance on a series of tasks often depends on the order in which the tasks are assigned. Order effects can confound experiment results when different orders are systematically (and inadvertently) associated with treatment and control conditions. A set of exam problems might be completed more quickly in one order than another, because one problem might prepare you for another but not vice versa. So if a control group of students is presented test problems in a "good" order and the treatment group gets the problems in a "bad" order, then a positive effect of treatment might be washed out by the effect of order; or, if the treatment group gets the "good" order, the effect of treatment (which could be zero) might appear larger than it is.

Treatment Interaction Effects. The term *interaction* refers to the fact that treatment can affect people differently depending on the subject's characteristics. Potential threats to external validity include the interaction between treatment and any of the following: selection, history, and testing.

SAMPLING: SELECTING SUBJECTS

Sampling refers to selecting subjects for the study. The sample comes from the population or the entire pool of possible subjects. In a classroom where the entire population is relatively small, testing all subjects may be simple. However, it is not possible to test an intervention on every new baby who is born, or every person diagnosed with heart failure or all adults with dementia. In this case, a smaller group or sample of the target population is gathered and tested and then inferences are made that are representative of the population. For a sample to be representative, it must resemble the entire population in as many ways as possible, but particularly with regard to the variables that are being studied or any known factors that might influence those variables (Burns & Grove, 2009). A study sample is found using either random (probability sampling) or nonrandom (nonprobability) methods.

Probability sampling, or *random sampling*, refers to the potential for any member of the population to be included in the study, making the sample representative of the population at large. *Randomization* means subjects are allocated by chance to one of the study groups. It characterizes a process of selection in which each person or entity in a study has an equal chance of being chosen for either the experimental (intervention) group or the control group. Random sampling can be simple, clustered, or stratified. Simple random sampling can be achieved by tossing a coin, throwing a die, pulling a name from a box that contains all potential subjects' names, or using a list of random numbers. This type of sampling can lead to an uneven number of participants in each group. To avert imbalances, random samples can also be stratified when some variables are known to be representative of the population, such as disease severity or gender (Figure 8.1). Cluster sampling assumes use of a naturally occurring group. Cluster sampling involves dividing the entire population (a state or a hospital) into clusters (zip code or nursing units) and then

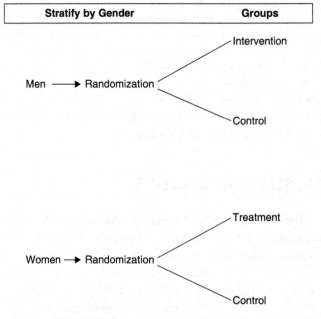

FIGURE 8.1 Stratified sampling.

using techniques of simple random sampling within each cluster. The primary difference between cluster sampling and stratified sampling is that when using a cluster, the entire cluster is studied. When stratifying, a random sample is taken from within each stratum. Data analysis is done by the cluster, for example, the results from the entire nursing unit, or by strata, for example, separate analysis for the men's group and the women's group. Cluster sampling can reduce the cost of the study; however, it is less precise than stratified sampling.

Nonprobability sampling does not involve a random selection of subjects. Rather, subjects are chosen based on their availability (or convenience) rather than their degree of representativeness of the population. Examples of nonprobability sampling include (Cochran, 2007):

■ Convenience sampling, in which subjects are chosen based on their ease of access, such as a group of friends or students in one classroom.
■ Snowball sampling, which involves a process of referral. One subject is selected, who then refers a friend, and the first friend refers a second, and so forth.
■ Purposive sampling, which is based on judgment, as the researcher chooses the sample based on some predetermined characteristics.
■ Quota sampling, which allows the researcher to choose any subject as long as a quota is met, for example, 60% of people in the study must be over age 50 years.

An interventional study can also be blinded. *Blinding* means to mask or hide something about the study or the intervention that might cause a bias in the study. For example, when testing the effectiveness of a drug on pain (vs. a placebo), the patient can be blinded as to what group the person is in (intervention or control). This is known as single-blind testing. If a study were to be double blind, then both the patient and the researcher would be blinded as to group assignment. Double-blind interventions decrease chance. Random assignment of subjects to the experimental and control groups is a critical part of any double-blind research design. The identity of the subjects in each of the groups is kept secured by a third person. A triple-blind study is an extension of the double-blind design with the addition that the assessor is also blinded. The assessor is simply given data from patients who are in group 1 or group 2 (Holly, Salmond, & Saimbert, 2012).

The number of subjects needed in a study can be determined by a power analysis. This statistical procedure is used to establish the number of required subjects needed in a study to show a significant difference at the study's level of significance. There are two web-based programs that can help in determining an adequate sample size:

- StatPages.net: This site provides links to a number of online power calculators:statpages.org/#Power
- G-Power: This site provides a downloadable power analysis program: www.psycho.uni-duesseldorf.de/abteilungen/aap/gpower3

ANALYZING RESULTS

A statistic represents a numerical version of information ranging from simple computations, such as determining the mean of a distribution, to the more complex determination of an effect size. There are two major types of statistics: descriptive statistics and inferential statistics. Descriptive statistics use numbers to describe a known data set. For example, the average length of stay for patients with heart failure in the past 2 years would be a descriptive statistic, as we are using all of the patients with a diagnosis of heart failure during that time period. Inferential statistics are used to draw conclusions about a population. Inferential statistics can be used for estimation or prediction, for example, the differences in test scores before and after use of simulated clinical laboratory activities. The specific statistical test used to analyze data depends on the type of the study and the level of data collected, for example (Tables 8.3 and 8.4):

TABLE 8.3

LEVELS OF MEASUREMENT

Level	Characteristics	Examples
Ratio	Magnitude Equal intervals Absolute zero	Age Height Weight Percentage
Interval	Magnitude Equal intervals	Temperature
Ordinal	Magnitude	Likert scale
Nominal	None	Names Lists

TABLE 8.4

DATA ANALYSIS

Type of Data Analysis	Statistical Test to Use
Description	Mean, standard deviation
One-group comparison	*t*-test
Two-group comparison, unpaired	Unpaired *t*-test
Two-group comparison, paired	Paired *t*-test
Three-or-more-groups comparison, unmatched	ANOVA (one way)
Three-or-more-groups comparison, matched	ANOVA (repeated measures)
Associations or relationships	Pearson correlation
Prediction	Regression ANOVA, analysis of variance.

■ Type of Study

Description (association): Correlations, factor analysis, path analysis
Explanation (prediction): Regression, logistic regression, discriminant analysis
Intervention (group differences): *t*-test, ANOVA (analysis of variance), MANOVA (multivariate analysis of variance), chi-square

■ Level of Data

Nominal: Chi-square, logistic regression
Dichotomous: Logistic regression
Ordinal: Chi-square
Interval/Ratio: Correlation

The results of statistical testing determine the significance of the findings. *Significance* refers to the level of confidence in the results of a study. In other words, if we want to be 95% confident in our results, we set the significance level at .05 (or 5%). If we want to be 99% confident, our significance level is .01. If statistics estimate that there is 10% error and the study is set at a .05 level, the results of the study would be stated as "not significant." In this case, the null hypothesis would be accepted (Holly et al., 2012). See Box 8.3 for online resources to assist in data analysis.

BOX 8.3

ONLINE RESOURCES FOR ANALYZING DATA

The Statistical Decision Tree: www.microsiris.com/Statistical%20Decision%20Tree/how_many_variables.htm

Selecting Statistics: www.socialresearchmethods.net/selstat/ssstart.htm

Interactive Statistical Tutorial: statpages.org/javasta4.html#Demos

WRITING THE RESEARCH REPORT

Research reports of quantitative findings from interventional studies are organized using a consistent pattern : title page, abstract, introduction, methods, results, discussion, references, appendices, and author note. The CONSORT statement, which stands for Consolidated Standards of Reporting Trials, can provide a guideline for preparing the final report (www.consort-statement.org).

Title. The title of a research report provides a brief summary of the report and should be no longer than 10 to 12 words.

Abstract. The abstract is the second page of the research report. It contains a short 200- to 300-word summary of the study, is one paragraph in length, and contains no references. It follows the major headings of the research report.

Main Document. The main body of the paper has four sections:

- **Introduction**. The purpose of the introduction is to introduce the reader to the topic and discuss the background of the issue at hand. The introduction also contains a review of the literature, which describes the current state of the topic that was investigated, the study objectives, and hypotheses proposed.
- **Methods**. The Methods section is second and refers to the procedures used to conduct the research. The study design setting, sample, recruitment strategies, randomization methods, subject demographics, and pilot test results should be described in enough detail to allow transparency for replication.
- **Results**. In this section the types of statistical tests used are described and results presented. Charts, tables, and graphs are

often included here. The Results section should address whether or not the null hypothesis was accepted or rejected.

■ **Discussion**. This section allows the researcher to describe the study and its implications and to suggest areas for further research on the topic. Limitations of the study are also included here.

References. This section contains all the literature cited in the report. Nothing else should be included here..

Appendices. If used, appendices are included at the end of the paper. Appendices should contain only material that is relevant and that assists readers in understanding the study.

CONCLUSIONS

Because nursing is a practice discipline, an understanding of how particular interventions work and in what context they work best can inform the dilemmas of practice and improve patient care guided by the results of clinical interventional research findings.

■ QUESTION FOR DISCUSSION

The households in two areas of a large urban city are sampled to determine the level of physical activity of those living in the two areas. The areas are stratified into high rent and low rent . There are 100 households in the high-rent area and 900 in the low-rent area. Discuss the type of sampling that should be used for this study, the data you would collect, and how data would be analyzed.

■ REFLECTIVE EXERCISE

1. Select a program that has been implemented where you work, such as a smoking-cessation program, an employee wellness program, or an AIDS prevention program. Determine:

   ■ The intervention specifications for the program
   ■ Key fidelity issues
   ■ Data used to determine the program's success
   ■ How human subjects were protected

EXAMPLES OF INTERVENTIONAL STUDIES

Effectiveness of Recruitment and Retention Strategies in a Pregnant Adolescent Nutrition Intervention Study

An important step to meeting the healthcare needs of pregnant adolescents is to conduct research studies that generate reliable and accurate data. However, recruitment and retention of pregnant adolescents into research is challenging and time intensive. This study reported the strategies used to recruit and retain pregnant adolescents into a nutrition-focused intervention study. A quasi-experimental, one-group, preintervention, postintervention, 6-week postintervention repeated-measures study was conducted among inner-city pregnant adolescents. The intervention involved pregnant adolescents' participation in an educational workshop. A total of four workshops were conducted over 14 months. Data were collected immediately after the intervention and 6 weeks following the intervention. The use of texting reminders and pregnant adolescent–related incentives that included gift bags and baby items were effective recruitment and retention strategies. Despite designing the recruitment strategies and using a developmentally tailored workshop, an adequate sample was unable to be recruited and retained for this study. A major barrier in developing evidence-based care practices to promote the health of these young mothers and their children involves recruiting and retaining them in research studies.

Reference

Wise, N. J., & Cantrell, M. A. (2018). Effectiveness of recruitment and retention strategies in a pregnant adolescent nutrition intervention study. *Journal of Advanced Nursing*. Epub ahead of print September 5. doi:10.1111/jan.13840

HEALTH PROMOTION IN SCHOOL-AGED HISPANIC CHILDREN THROUGH A CULTURALLY APPROPRIATE NUTRITION AND EXERCISE FAMILY-SCHOOL PROGRAM

Purpose/Objectives: The purpose of the project was to promote lifestyle changes for health in Hispanic school children and their families related to diet and physical activity. The specific objectives for this project were to:

1. Maintain or improve participants' preintervention clinical assessment findings.
2. Increase caregivers' knowledge of healthy nutrition and physical activity.
3. Analyze caregivers' dietary patterns based on national guidelines.
4. Promote development of consistent healthy patterns of nutrition and physical activity.

(continued)

HEALTH PROMOTION IN SCHOOL-AGED HISPANIC CHILDREN THROUGH A CULTURALLY APPROPRIATE NUTRITION AND EXERCISE FAMILY-SCHOOL PROGRAM (*CONTINUED*)

Hypotheses: (a) Participation in the educational program increases caregivers' practices of healthy nutrition; (b) participation in the educational program increases the level of caregivers' physical activity; and (c) participation in the educational program leads to reduction in weight for caregivers, improvement in body mass index (BMI)-for-age for children, and improvement in blood pressure levels of both caregivers and children.

Methodology: The research design was quantitative pretest–posttest using a demographic survey, the Health Promoting Lifestyle Profile II (HPLP II) tool, and pre- and postclinical assessments. A culturally and linguistically appropriate educational program was designed to promote family-oriented healthy nutrition and physical activity practices. Preliminary assessment of the neighborhood, school meals, and Hispanic family food and physical activity practices guided the development of the educational program. The windshield survey of the neighborhood surrounding the project setting was aimed to identify barriers to healthy nutrition and current levels of participation in physical activity by residents. The assessment included a review of neighborhood safety, parks and recreational facilities, transportation, and food establishments. Interviews with school lunch aides provided a preliminary assessment of students' food patterns and preferences. Recommendations for an improvement to the lunch experience included the following: a less rushed atmosphere, maintaining proper temperature of food, offering of ethnic foods, and finding creative ways to have children try fruits and vegetables. An interview with the director of food services provided an overview of federal mandates for school breakfasts and lunches. Children's free access to food, amount of time spent watching television, and participation in physical activity were addressed with caregivers during the parent–teacher meetings. The educational program designed for the project (the intervention) incorporated the findings of the preliminary assessment.

The program was implemented weekly for 10 weeks on consecutive Saturdays. The weekend schedule was chosen to accommodate the family-oriented participation in activities common among Hispanics. Each session consisted of 2.5 hours divided into two component parts: (a) 90 minutes on promoting healthy diet and lifestyle behaviors for the family and developing a family approach to incorporate traditional Hispanic food preferences into healthy cooking practices, and (b) 60 minutes of low-impact aerobic activity for the family. Areas of special interest to Hispanic families, such as dancing and using popular Hispanic music, were used. All learning activities were conducted in English and Spanish, which included lecture presentation and fun activities such as a healthy food store tour, family health/nutrition bingo, and family physical activities.

Caregivers kept a daily log of their food intake and physical activity. Analysis of the weekly food and activity logs was given to each caregiver. Discussion of the analysis was done in a focus group format with individual counseling

(*continued*)

HEALTH PROMOTION IN SCHOOL-AGED HISPANIC CHILDREN THROUGH A CULTURALLY APPROPRIATE NUTRITION AND EXERCISE FAMILY-SCHOOL PROGRAM (*CONTINUED*)

if needed. Findings were reported to participants as aggregate data. Pre- and posteducational program assessments were done using one instrument, the HPLP II, and clinical assessment of weight, BMI, and blood pressures.

Participants: Participants in the study were a convenience sample drawn from parents of school children attending one elementary school located in a predominantly Hispanic community. The sample was composed of 14 caregivers and their school-aged children. The criteria for caregiver eligibility included the following: (a) self-identified as Hispanic, (b) having a child enrolled in the public school in preschool through fifth grade, (c) living in the same household as the child, (d) responsible for preparing or purchasing food for the child's household, (5) no self-reported medical condition that would prohibit physical activity, (6) agreement to complete the 10-week project implementation period. Participation in this intervention presented no identified risks. An advanced practice nurse was available at all times throughout the intervention. A written consent form was offered. All participants were able to read and write. A written assent form was offered to all children.

Findings: Hypotheses 1 and 2 were supported by paired sample *t*-tests on the pre- and postmeans of caregivers on the HPLP Nutrition and Physical Activity subscales. With regard to Hypothesis 3, significant difference in the pre- and post-BMI and pre- and postsystolic blood pressure of school-aged children were found through the paired samples *t*-test. In contrast, the *t*-test comparison on the caregivers was not significant. However, comparison of means in all parameters—weight, BMI, diastolic and systolic blood pressure—revealed a change in the means from higher preintervention to lower postintervention means. It is possible that because the sample was small and the mean differences were not pronounced, statistical significance was not achieved.

Conclusion: The study attempted to determine the outcomes of an educational intervention on knowledge and practices of healthy nutrition and physical activity in a group of Hispanic school-aged children and their caregivers. Implementation of a cultural and linguistic educational program is effective in changing nutritional and physical activity practices that can impact on health status of adults and children. The study demonstrated a successful model for recruiting and retaining Hispanic participants in a combined nutrition and physical activity intervention. The intervention was an important first step in designing an ongoing multidisciplinary nutrition and physical activity program and points to the need for continued research to decrease health disparities in Hispanics.

Reference

Echevarria, M. (2011). Health promotion in school-aged Hispanic children through a culturally appropriate nutrition and exercise family—School program. In C. Holly, S. Salmond, & M. Saimbert (Eds.), *Scholarly inquiry and the DNP capstone* (pp. 101–103). New York, NY: Springer Publishing.

■ SUGGESTED READINGS

Harkness, J., Lederer, S., & Wikler, D. (2001). Laying ethical foundations for clinical research. *Bulletin of the World Health Organization, 79*(4), 365–372.

Lopez, L. M., Tolley, E. E., Grimes, D. A., & Chen-Mok, M. (2009). Theory-based interventions for contraception. *Cochrane Database of Systematic Review, 2009*(3), CD007249. doi:10.1002/14651858.CD007249.pub2

Naylor, M. (2003). Nursing intervention research and quality of care: Influencing the future of healthcare. *Nursing Research, 52*(6), 380–385. doi:10.1097/00006199-200311000-00005

Whittemore, R., & Grey, M. (2002). The systematic development of nursing interventions. *Journal of Nursing Scholarship, 34*(2), 115–120. doi:10.1111/j.1547-5069.2002.00115.x

■ REFERENCES

Burns, N., & Grove, S. (2009). *The practice of nursing research* (6th ed.). Philadelphia, PA: Saunders/Elsevier.

Cochran, W. (2007). *Sampling techniques*. New York, NY: Wiley.

Cohen, P. (1995). *Order effects*. Retrieved April 20, 2013, http://www.cs.colostate.edu/~howe/EMAI/ch3/node11.html

Dumas, J., Lynch, A., Laughlin, J., Smith, E., & Prinz, R. (2001). Promoting intervention fidelity: Conceptual issues, methods, and preliminary results from the EARLY ALLIANCE prevention trial. *American Journal of Preventive Medicine, 20*(1), 38–47. doi:10.1016/S0749-3797(00)00272-5

Echevarria, M. (2011). Health promotion in school-aged Hispanic children through a culturally appropriate nutrition and exercise family—School program. In C. Holly, S. Salmond, & M. Saimbert (Eds.), *Scholarly inquiry and the DNP capstone* (pp. 101–103). New York, NY: Springer Publishing.

Fleury, J., & Sidani, S. (2012). Using theory to guide intervention research. In B. Melnyk, & D. Morrison-Beedy (Eds.), *Intervention research: Designing, conducting, analyzing, funding* (pp. 11–36). New York, NY: Springer Publishing.

Forbes, A. (2009). Clinical intervention research in nursing. *International Journal of Nursing Studies, 46*, 557–568. doi:10.1016/j.ijnurstu.2008.08.012

Hoffman, A. J., Brintnall, R. A., Brown, J. K., Eye, A. V., Jones, L. W., Alderink, G., . . . Vanotteren, G. M. (2013). Too sick not to exercise: Using a 6-week, home-based exercise intervention for cancer-related fatigue self-management for postsurgical non-small cell lung cancer patients. *Cancer Nursing, 36*(3), 175–188. doi:10.1097/NCC.0b013e31826c7763

Holly, C., Salmond, S., & Saimbert, M. (2012). *Comprehensive systematic review for advanced nursing practice*. New York, NY: Springer Publishing.

Ibrahim, K., May, C. R., Patel, H. P., Baxter, M., Sayer, A. A., & Roberts, H. C. (2018). Implementation of grip strength measurement in medicine for older people wards as part of routine admission assessment: Identifying facilitators and barriers using a theory-led intervention. *BMC Geriatrics, 18*(1), 79. doi:10.1186/s12877-018-0768-5

Mathey, M., Vanneste, V., Graaf, C., deGroot, L., & van Staeren, W. (2001). Health of improved meal ambiance in a Dutch nursing home: A 1-year intervention study. *Preventive Medicine, 32*(5), 416–423. doi:10.1006/pmed.2001.0816

Melynk, B., & Cole, R. (2011). Generating evidence through quantitative research. In B. Melnyk & E. Fineout-Overholt (Eds.), *Evidence based practice in nursing and healthcare: A guide to best practice* (2nd ed, pp. 397–434). Philadelphia, PA: Wolters Kluwer/Lippicott Williams & Wilkins.

Melnyk, B., Morrison-Beedy, D., & Moore, S. (2012). The nuts and bolts of designing intervention studies. In B. Melnyk & D. Morrison-Beedy (Eds.), *Intervention research: Designing, conducting, analyzing, funding* (pp. 37–63). New York, NY: Springer Publishing.

Meraviglia, M., Stuifbergen, A., Parsons, D., & Morgans, S. (2013). Health promotion for cancer survivors: Adaptation and implementation of an intervention. *Holistic Nursing Practice, 27*(3), 140–147. doi:10.1097/HNP.0b013e31828a0988

Muntlin, A., Carlsso, M., Safwenberg, U., & Gunningberg, L. (2011). Outcomes of a nurse-initiated intravenous analgesic protocol for abdominal pain in an emergency department: A quasi-experimental study. *International Journal of Nursing Studies, 48*(1), 13–23. doi:10.1016/j.ijnurstu.2010.06.003

National Institutes of Health. (2013). *e-Source: Behavioral and social science research.* Washington, DC: Author. Retrieved from http://www.esourceresearch.org/tabid/36/Default.aspx

Navidian, A., & Bahari, F. (2013). The impact of mixed, hope and forgiveness-focused marital counselling on interpersonal cognitive distortions of couples filing for divorce. *Journal of Psychiatric and Mental Health Nursing, 21,* 658–666. doi:10.1111/jpm.12058

Paradis, V., Cossette, S., Smith, N., Heppell, S., & Guertin, M. C. (2010). The efficacy of a motivational nursing intervention based on the stages of change on self-care in heart failure patients. *Journal of Cardiovascular Nursing, 25*(2), *130–141. doi:10.1097/JCN.0b013e3181c52497*

Santacroce, S., Maccarelli, L., & Grey, M. (2004). Intervention fidelity. *Nursing Research, 53*(1), 63–66. doi:10.1097/00006199-200401000-00010

Weatherspoon, D., & Wyatt, T. (2012). Testing computer-based simulation to enhance clinical judgment skills in senior nursing students. *Nursing Clinics of North America, 47*(4), 481–491. doi:10.1016/j.cnur.2012.07.002

Wise, N. J., & Cantrell, M. A. (2018). Effectiveness of recruitment and retention strategies in a pregnant adolescent nutrition intervention study. *Journal of Advanced Nursing.* Epub ahead of print September 5. doi:10.1111/jan.13840

Wyatt, T., & Hauenstein, E. (2008). Pilot: An online asthma intervention for school aged children. *Journal of School Nursing, 24*(3), 145–150. doi:10.1177/1059840522334455

Zhou, Y., Liao, J., Feng, F., Ji, M., Zhao, C., & Wang, X. (2018). Effects of a nurse-led phone follow-up education program based on the self-efficacy among patients with cardiovascular disease. *Journal of Cardiovascular Nursing, 33*(1), E15–E23. doi:10.1097/JCN.0000000000000414

CHAPTER 9

Systematic Review

▦ OBJECTIVES

At the end of this chapter, you will be able to:

- Differentiate among the types of systematic review.
- Delineate the benefits of a systematic review.
- Outline the steps in a systematic review.
- Describe new and emerging methods of systematic review.

▦ KEY CONCEPTS

- A systematic review is a secondary analysis of existing data.
- Systematic reviews bring the same level of rigor to the research process as is found in primary studies.
- Systematic reviews can inform us about what is known, what is not known, and what needs to be known.
- Systematic reviews may be conducted using quantitative evidence, qualitative evidence, or both.
- Systematic reviews provide a balanced and impartial summary of findings with consideration given to the strengths and weaknesses of included studies.
- The findings of a systematic review can provide the foundation for primary research.

INTRODUCTION

Systematic reviews are based in population health, where every person is different and unique but similar enough so that we can determine what

BOX 9.1

BENEFITS OF A SYSTEMATIC REVIEW

A clear question guides the review.

Large amounts of information that have been critically appraised to be rigorous are collapsed into a manageable, usable form.

It provides a clearer, less biased understanding because of the systematic process used in the review as well as the checks and balances of two researchers.

A systematic review increases the strength and generalizability/transferability of the findings, because they are derived from a broader range of populations, settings, circumstances, treatment variations, and study designs.

It minimizes bias from random and systematic error.

A systematic review pools and synthesizes existing information for decisions about clinical care, economics, future research designs, and policy formation.

It assesses consistencies and provides explanations for inconsistencies of relationships across studies.

A systematic review increases confidence in the cause-and-effect relationships suggested.

Systematic review increases confidence in conclusions drawn.

It increases the likelihood of results being used in clinical practice.

It provides a format for ongoing updates of new evidence.

Systematic reviews helps practitioners keep up to date with overwhelming quantities of medical literature.

Source: Holly, C., Salmond, S., & Saimbert, M. (2012). *Comprehensive systematic review for advanced nursing practice* (p. 14). New York, NY: Springer Publishing. Reprinted with permission.

works best overall and under what circumstances best outcomes can be achieved (Holly, Salmond, & Saimbert, 2016). A systematic review is a descriptive method of research in which the subjects or informants in the study are published or unpublished primary studies, rather than human subjects. In other words, systematic reviews research information, not human subjects. The word *systematic* refers to a logical and orderly approach that mirrors the process used in primary studies. Systematic reviews allow practitioners to make point-of-care decisions based on the best available evidence for a focused clinical question. When making healthcare decisions, it is preferred practice to look at a body of evidence rather than the results of one study (Chalmers, 2006). The benefits of a systematic review are many (see Box 9.1), including:

■ Providing reliable evidential summaries of completed research that are more powerful than the results of a single study

- Providing outcome data that can be used in policy decisions
- Clarifying existing data to avoid duplication in research studies
- Helping practitioners stay current in the face of overwhelming quantities of health-related literature

TYPES OF REVIEWS

There are two basic types of systematic review: a quantitative meta-analysis, which uses the results of randomized controlled trials (RCTs) or observational studies, and a qualitative meta-synthesis, which uses the results of phenomenology, grounded theory, ethnography, action research, or other qualitative methods. Meta-analysis and meta-synthesis are umbrella terms for the way in which data are analyzed within a systematic review.

Meta-Analysis

Meta-analysis is statistical synthesis of data that are pooled for analysis from a set of similar studies on the same topic. The general aim of a meta-analysis is to estimate the effect of interventions or treatments under a given single set of assumptions and conditions. The term *meta-analysis* was originally coined by Glass (1978), who stated, "The term is a bit grand, but it is precise and apt. . . . Meta-analysis refers to the analysis of analyses" (p. 3).

Meta-analysis is a systematic investigation of effect sizes and the exploration of their variation across studies. An effect size is a quantitative measure of the strength of a phenomenon, as in the correlation of hypertension and a high-salt diet. A large effect size indicates a stronger effectunless the effect size is an odds ratio. For instance, a meta-analysis may be conducted using the results of several clinical trials of a drug treatment or a self-care management educational intervention in an effort to obtain a better understanding of how well the treatment or intervention worked. A summary of the pooled results, called an *effect size*, is provided. In addition to providing an effect size, a meta-analysis can identify patterns among study results or sources of disagreement among those results.

A meta-analysis examines two general areas:

1. *The strength and direction of the findings.* The central purpose of a meta-analysis is to test the relationship between two variables and determine how one affects the other. Summary statistics

identify whether X (e.g., obesity) affects Y (e.g., walking) by summarizing significance levels, effect sizes (the measure of the difference of two treatment effects), and/or confidence intervals.

2. *The variability among the studies in the review.* There will always be variation in a meta-analysis. The question is whether the degree of variability is significantly different than what we would expect by chance alone (heterogeneity). Cochran's Q measures heterogeneity. It is calculated as the weighted sum of squared differences between individual study effects and the pooled effect across studies. Q is presented as a chi-square statistic with k (number of studies) minus 1 degree of freedom. The Q test only informs about the presence versus the absence of heterogeneity. It does not report the extent of heterogeneity or any reasons for the heterogeneity. The I^2 (I square) index is available to report on extent. The I^2 index complements the Q test. If there is significant heterogeneity (variability), the next step is to look for moderating variables that can explain the variability. In other words, does the effect of X (obesity) on Y (walking) differ with moderator variables (gym membership, incentives)?

Often an individual clinical trial fails to show any significant difference between two methods of treatment or two different interventions. However, when the results of individual studies are combined, significant benefits of one treatment over the other can be realized. For example, Bahekar, Singh, Saha, Molnar, and Arora (2007) reported that previous studies have shown conflicting results as to whether periodontitis (PD) is associated with increased risk of coronary heart disease (CHD). They conducted a systematic review and meta-analysis of five prospective cohort studies (86,092 patients) and found that individuals with PD had a 1.14 times higher risk of developing CHD than the controls (relative risk: 1.14, 95% confidence interval [CI]: 1.074–1.213, $p < .001$), indicating that both the prevalence and incidence of CHD are significantly increased in PD and PD may be a risk factor for CHD.

Studies used in a meta-analysis can be experimental or descriptive, although RCTs are preferred. An RCT is a carefully controlled clinical trial that studies the effect of a therapy (intervention or treatment) on actual patients. Attention is paid to randomization to study group (experimental or control group), blinding, and bias.

Observational studies can also be used in a review. These include cohort studies, case-control studies, case series, or case reports. Cohort studies follow a large population over time. Subjects have the same condition (e.g., cancer) or receive the same treatment over time (e.g., chemotherapy). Comparisons are made with another group without the condition or treatment being studied. Case-control studies are about patients who already have a specific condition (e.g., HIV/AIDS). Patient outcomes are compared with those who do not have this condition. Medical records and patient historical recall are used to collect data. Case series and case reports are narratives about the treatment of individual or groups of patients. There are no controls or comparisons for case series or case reports (Holly et al., 2016).

Meta-analyses are conducted using a predetermined model for analysis, either a fixed-effect model or a random-effect model. A fixed-effect model provides a weighted average of the study estimates in which the weights are the inverse variance of the study estimate. Consequently, studies with a larger sample size are given greater weight in the analysis regardless of the significance of findings. In other words, larger studies dominate the analysis. Smaller studies, though significant in their findings, can be ignored. Fixed-effect models are useful when there is certainty that the underlying effects are the same for all studies. As this is rarely the case in health-related research, findings may be difficult to interpret, and have a very narrow confidence interval (lack of precision). To allow for the differences between health-related studies (heterogeneity), a random-effect model should be used. In this model, the weight of each study is redistributed, and an unweighted average for the effect size is determined across studies, equalizing the studies regardless of sample size (Box 9.2).

A new model, called a *quality model*, is gaining popularity. In this model, study quality is used in combination with study weight. This allows the methodological quality of a study, determined during the appraisal process, to be used along with study findings when analyzing results. In other words, if a study is of good quality and other studies are of poor quality, a proportion of their quality-adjusted weights is mathematically redistributed, giving the good study more weight toward the overall effect size. As studies increase in quality, redistribution becomes progressively smaller and ceases when all studies are of perfect quality (Doi & Thalib, 2008). A software program is available to conduct this analysis as a free add-on to Excel (MetaXL, 2012).

Meta-Synthesis

Meta-synthesis refers to the aggregation or interpretation of findings from qualitative studies. The intent of meta-synthesis is to bring together findings, categorize these findings into groups on the basis of similarity in meaning, and aggregate or interpret these to generate a set of statements that adequately represent the combined studies (synthesized

BOX 9.2

HETEROGENEITY

Heterogeneity is about clinical variation. In health-related research this can be due to, for example, differences in the sample (age, gender, comorbidities), study site (hospital, nursing home, clinic, home care agency), or condition (severity of illness).

The chi-squared test provides an indication of the significance of heterogeneity, but it does not measure it. A measurement index for heterogeneity is provided by I^2, a percentage of the chi-squared statistic that is not explained by the variation within the studies. It represents the percentage of the total variation, which is due to variation between studies.

To interpret I^2:

I^2 = 0% = no heterogeneity
I^2 = 25% = low heterogeneity
I^2 = 50% = moderate heterogeneity
I^2 = 75% = high heterogeneity

In this example, I^2 = 71%, p = .003, shows that there is a high level of heterogeneity and the chi-square result determines that this is significantly high. In this case, a determination has to be made as to whether there is too much variation to pool the studies and a narrative review should therefor be conducted.

Source: Higgins, J. P. T., & Thompson, S. G. (2002). Quantifying heterogeneity in a meta-analysis. Statistics in Medicine, 21, 1539–1558. doi:10.1002/sim.1186; Higgins, J. P. T., Thompson, S. G., Deeks, J. J., & Altman, D. G. (2003). Measuring inconsistency in meta-analyses. British Medical Journal, 327, 557–560. doi:10.1136/bmj.327.7414.557

findings). These statements then can be used as a basis for evidence-based practice (Holly et al., 2016).

Studies used in meta-synthesis include:

■ Phenomenology, which presents the lived experiences and the meaning of those experiences from the viewpoint of the subject and aims to provide a greater depth of understanding about the experiences in people's lives
■ Grounded theory, which explores social processes among humans and generates new theoretical constructs that illuminate human behavior in a social world
■ Ethnography, which attempts to show how people in a specific culture or subculture make sense of their experiences and realities

- Action research, which uses a specific process to improve a situation
- Qualitative descriptive studies, which provide an uncomplicated description of events using the words of interviewed subjects with little to no interpretation

The findings drawn from these various methods are translated one into another using colloquial, rather than word-for-word, translation, "creating a broader and deeper understanding of the phenomenon" under investigation (Holly et al., 2012, p. 224). *Translating* indicates that similar concepts are identified in each individual study, although they may be expressed differently. These concepts are combined in ways that go beyond the question originaly posed. This is primarily done through meta-aggregation, meta-ethnography, or a qualitative descriptive meta-summary (Table 9.1).

Meta-aggregation is the summing, or integration of findings, from primary studies that allows a comprehensive summary of statements. For example, Vaismoradi, Skär, Söderberg, and Bondas (2016) integrated the experiences of older persons' meaning of pain, how pain was experienced, and how it was managed in nursing homes, based on

TABLE 9.1

TYPES OF META-SYNTHESIS	
Meta-ethnography	An interpretive synthesis (interpretation of interpretations) that arises from comparative translation. It is not limited to ethnographic studies.
Meta-aggregation	The aggregation or synthesis of findings to generate a set of statements which represent that aggregation by assembling the findings according to their quality rating and categorizing these findings on the basis of similarity in meaning. These categories are then subjected to a meta-synthesis in order to produce a single comprehensive set of synthesized findings that can be used as a basis for evidence-based practice.
Meta-summary (descriptive meta-synthesis)	An approach to synthesize reports of primary qualitative studies containing findings in the form of topical or thematic summaries or surveys of the data the researcher has collected. There is little interpretation involved.

Source: Holly, C., Salmond, S., & Saimbert, M. (2016). *Comprehensive systematic review for advanced nursing practice* (2nd ed.). New York, NY: Springer Publishing.

the perspectives and experiences of all involved in pain management. Three themes were identified: identity of pain, recognition of pain, and response to pain.

In contrast, meta-ethnography is a method used to deduce new meaning, rather than to reinterpret original meanings. Findings are not aggregated but rather are analyzed to create new knowledge and conceptual models of understanding. For example, Ho and Chiang (2015) developed a schema for the optimism of the migration and a general framework of motivated psychosocial and behavioral adaptation was proposed. This meta-ethnography also revealed the vulnerabilities of migrant nurses in the process of acculturation and socialization.

A meta-summary presents findings in the form of topical or thematic summaries. Little interpretation is involved. To illustrate, using a meta-summary, Childress (2013) condensed themes on the lived experiences and coping mechanisms among culturally diverse domestic violence survivors. These themes include:

- The effects of violence
- The cyclical nature of violence
- Normalizing and tolerating violence
- The strength and resilience of victims
- Barriers to help-seeking
- The role of substance use in domestic violence

STEPS IN A SYSTEMATIC REVIEW

Similar to primary studies, systematic reviews have a specific methodology to follow (Box 9.3). Steps in the systematic review process include:

Formulate a Focused Clinical Question

A focused question is one that is useful to practitioners, leads to a change in practice based on new evidence, or increases confidence in usual care (Kitchenham, 2004). Questions for a systematic review must be carefully considered, as too broad a question will result in an unmanageable amount of papers to review. Too narrow a question could result in a meaningless exercise, as the phenomenon of interest may not be captured. Generally, one is recommended to begin with a tight focus and make changes as needed to identify whether there are appropriate and sufficient papers for inclusion in the review (Holly et al., 2016). Typically, review questions focus on interventions or therapy, etiology

BOX 9.3

STEPS IN A META-ANALYSIS

1. Formulate a focused clinical question.
2. Determine key words and phrases. Search the literature.
3. Select studies:

   - Critically appraise each study.
   - Include unpublished studies to avoid publication bias.

4. Determine summary measures for extraction:

   - Differences (discrete data)
   - Means (continuous data)
   - Use a data-extraction tool to extract all data

5. Choose a model for analysis:

   - Fixed-effect model

This model provides a weighted average of the study estimates. The sample size within each study determines how much weight is given to the study, which allows larger studies to dominate regardless of findings. This model is used when the intent is to generalize only to the review population.

   - Random-effect model

This model uses the confidence interval (a measure of precision) to determine the weight each study is given. This model should be used when the intent is to generalize to a larger population.

6. Interpret results and draw conclusions:

   - The conclusions drawn from a meta-analysis can be used as best practice recommendations, if appropriate.

Source: Adapted from Holly, C., & Slyer, J. (2013). Interpreting and using meta-analysis in clinical practice. *Orthopedic Nursing, 32*(2), 106–110.

or causation, diagnosis, prognosis, economics, or meaning (Table 9.2). A review question about what intervention or therapy works most effectively is best answered using RCTs. Questions of etiology or causation assist in identifying the likely causes of a condition. Diagnosis or diagnostic testing questions are concerned with how well a diagnostic test works, and questions of prognosis deal with how to estimate the patient's

TABLE 9.2

EXAMPLES OF SYSTEMATIC REVIEW QUESTIONS

Type of Review	Question Example	Best Study to Use in a Review
Intervention or therapy	What is the effect of telephone follow-up and counseling versus no follow-up in 90-day readmission rates for heart failure?	RCT Cohort Case control Case series
Etiology, screening, risk/harm	What are the risk factors for development of coronary artery disease in Asian Indians?	RCT Cohort Case control Case series
Diagnosis or diagnostic testing	What test works best for the diagnosis of TB?	Prospective comparison to a gold standard
Prognosis or prediction	Over the course of 2 years, what happens to patients diagnosed with a chronic disease?	Cohort study Case control Case series
Economics	What type of PICC line decreases cost and site infection in children on chemotherapy?	Cost-benefit Cost utilization Cost minimization
Meaning	What outcomes are most important to patients undergoing treatment for obesity?	Qualitative

PICC, peripherally inserted central catheter; RCT, randomized controlled trial; TB, tuberculosis.

likely clinical course over time and what complications are likely to occur. Cost underlies economic questions. Questions of meaning are about the experiences, perceptions, feelings, and opinions of the study participant regarding a particular topic or experience and use qualitative studies for review.

Well-formulated questions use the PICO format, in which:

P stands for *population, patients,* or *phenomenon of interest.*
I is used to describe the intervention or approach to be studied.
C is for *comparison* or main alternatives to the intervention to be studied.
O stands for *outcome.*

An example of a therapy question for a systematic review using this pneumonic is "In teenage boys (P) how effective is a peer counseling program (I) in reducing smoking (O)?" The comparison would be teenage boys who are not enrolled in the peer counseling program.

Systematic reviews of qualitative studies use a modified version of PICO, in which the C and the O are combined to denote context: PICo. For example, "How do family members (P) who witness an out-of-hospital cardiac resuscitation by emergency personnel (I) perceive the experience in the first month of grieving (Co)?" (Holly et al., 2016, p. 16).

Taking time to write the question will make searching for relevant studies for inclusion in the review easier and more timely, as the inclusion criteria should be evident in the question.

Find and Extract the Right Studies

Searching for the right studies to use for a systematic review is the equivalent of data collection in a primary study. The PICO question is used to determine the key words needed for searching. In the preceding example, "In teenage boys (P) how effective is a peer counseling program (I) in reducing smoking (O)?" the key words are *teenage boys*, *smoking*, and *peer counseling*. To broaden the search so that nothing is missed, alternative words or phrases should also be used, such as *adolescent boys* or *smoking reduction/smoking-cessation programs*. A concept map is useful in identifying all of the key words and their alternatives (Figure 9.1). RCTs (or other studies of effect) should also be an inclusion criteria, as this is an effectiveness review.

To conduct the search, select the databases to be used that best represent the field of the study (e.g., nursing, social work, psychology) or use other health-related databases. There is no set number of databases to search; however, the search should be as exhaustive as possible so that all relevant papers are found. Each database selected for searching has a short video introduction on how to use the database and how words are indexed. It is important to watch these before beginning

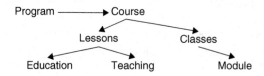

FIGURE 9.1 Concept map for *program*.

the search, as each database indexes differently. For example, the word *handwashing* may have been entered into a database as *handwashing*, *hand washing*, or *hand-washing*. When searching for nursing studies, the following databases are useful places to start:

1. Academic Search Premier
2. Medline (Medical Literature Analysis and Retrieval System Online)/PubMed
3. CINAHL (Cumulative Index to Nursing and Allied Health Literature) and pre-CINAHL
4. Embase
5. Web of Science
6. ClinicalTrials.gov

When conducting a systematic review, it is important to determine whether or not a review of the topic has already been done. A search of the Cochrane, Campbell, or Joanna Briggs libraries of systematic reviews or other review sites (Box 9.4) will help determine this. In the event a review on the topic has been found, it can be extended if the review is 3 to 5 or more years old. In this case, the review would need to be identified as an extension of the original work.

To decrease the bias associated with using only published studies in a systematic review, grey literature (unpublished) sites should also be searched. Searching the grey literature sites can provide conference

BOX 9.4

SYSTEMATIC REVIEW SITES

The Joanna Briggs Institute
www.joannabriggs.edu.au

The Cochrane Library
www.cochrane.org

The Campbell Collection
www.campbellcollection.org

PubMed Clinical Inquiry: Find Systematic Reviews
www.ncbi.nlm.nih.gov

Bandolier
www.medicine.ox.ac.uk/bandolier

The NHS Center for Reviews and Dissemination
www.york.ac.uk

proceedings, white papers, and other material useful to the review. These include:

- World Health Organization, Centers for Disease Control and Prevention, or state health departments
- The *Grey Literature Report*, a bimonthly publication of The New York Academy of Medicine Library
- National Technical Information Service (United States), the largest central resource for U.S. government-funded scientific, technical, engineering, and business-related information available today
- OAIster, a catalog of records representing open-access resources, including theses, technical reports and research papers, and digital items
- Google Scholar
- OpenGrey (formerly SIGLE), includes a collection of bibliographical references of graey literature produced in Europe
- NLM Gateway (National Library of Medicine) identifies studies and author contact information, particularly for clinical trials
- The Virginia Henderson Library of Sigma Theta Tau International and Magnet Conference Proceedings, provides abstract and author contact information

Other methods of searching for relevant studies include hand searching, use of personal contacts (circle of friends), and reviewing reference lists (harvesting). Hand searching involves identifying journals that are directly related to the focus of the review (e.g., *Pain and Analgesia Journal* for a study on pain management). This is a time-consuming but necessary task, as not all articles are indexed in electronic bibliographic databases. Personally contacting principal investigators of studies related to the review topic or other experts in the field can help identify unpublished or in-progress work. Each person contacted can also be asked to identify other persons who might have additional information (snowballing technique). Reviewing the reference lists of simple reviews of the literature and those papers retrieved for the review can also help identify additional sources that can be added to the review (Holly et al., 2016; Littell, Corcoran, & Pillai, 2008).

For each database searched, a record should be kept, which includes the date of the search, the title of the database (with URL), the range of dates searched, and the results of the search. The assistance of a research librarian with knowledge of the process of a systematic review would be an invaluable asset to a well-developed and documented search.

Appraising Studies

When an exhaustive search has been completed, the studies retrieved for the review must be appraised for methodological quality. As the purpose of a systematic review is to make recommendations for best practice and to establish whether or not the findings of primary research are consistent over time and for differing populations, the studies included in the review should be of the highest quality. A critical appraisal is done to determine the validity, value, and relevance to the particular clinical question under review. When appraising the validity of a study, attention to sources of potential bias, or threat, is essential. Threats include:

- Effects of repeated testing (pretest and posttest designs)
- Selection—Subjects who agree to participate in a study may be very different from those who refuse participation
- Mortality/attrition—Subjects withdraw from the study before completion and may be very different from the subjects who complete the study
- History—Events that occur during the conduct of the study may have influenced the treatment or the outcome; therefore, the treatment may not yield the same results at a different time
- Instrumentation—Use of the same test on multiple occasions may cue the subject to the hypothesis
- Performance—The fact that a subject is in a research study may result in behaviors that are not usual

There are several highly regarded tools that can be used for this appraisal, such as CASP (Critical Appraisal Skills Programme; www .sph.nhs.uk/what-we-do/public-health-workforce/resources/critical -appraisals-skills-programme) and Joanna Briggs Institute tools (joan-nabriggsinstitute.edu.au). There are different checklist tools with questions for the appraisal specific to the type of study being appraised, such as RCT, cohort, or case series or meaning. The checklists developed by the Joanna Briggs Institute include one for appraisal of economic studies.

To begin the appraisal, the basic questions to ask regarding any research study are:

- Has the research been conducted in such a way as to minimize bias? If so, what does the study show?
- What do the results mean for the particular patient or context in which a decision is being made (Burls, 2009)?

Questions for appraisal become more specific and focus on:

1. The clarity of the clinical question with regards to the population, intervention, and outcome (or phenomenon of interest in a qualitative systematic review)
2. The presence and description of explicit criteria for inclusion of subjects into the study
3. The match among the clinical question, study design, and data-collection and data-analysis methods
4. Evidence of any bias in the study, including selection bias (a biased distribution to groups), performance bias (different care or instructions provided that are not a part of study protocol), detection bias (uncovering group allocation), or attrition bias (lost to follow-up)

The major purpose of a critical appraisal is to select only those studies that are of the highest quality so that any recommendations made as a result of the systematic review are based on high-quality evidence. Studies retrieved for appraisal but then excluded should be reported along with the reason for exclusion. Reasons for exclusion should be related to methodology, rather than not meeting inclusion criteria.

Construct a Table of Evidence

A table of evidence is a chart that displays the characteristics of all the studies included in the systematic review (Table 9.3). Each study listed in the table of evidence should be graded as to its level of evidence. Not all evidence is of equal value. Regardless of which grading system is used, there are commonalities across the various grading systems. The highest level of evidence is agreed to be the RCT (referred to as *level I evidence*). Following this is evidence obtained from a controlled trial without randomization or evidence obtained from multiple time series with or without the intervention (referred to as *level II evidence*). The third (level III) level of evidence is obtained from observational studies, such as cohort or case-control study. The lowest grade of evidence (referred to as *level IV*) is the opinion of respected authorities, based on clinical experience, case studies, or reports of expert committees.

For reviews of effectiveness, confidence in the systematic review findings is determined by rating the findings using GRADE (Grading of Recommendations, Assessment, Development and Evaluations) and comparing these ratings. GRADE can rate the certainty of the evidence and specifically assesses methodological flaws within the component studies, consistency of results across different studies, generalizability

TABLE 9.3

TABLE OF EVIDENCE

Question: What is the impact of the synergy model on the nurse, patient, and system outcomes?

Source	Study Purpose	Method	Design/Level of Evidence	Variables	Results	Comment
Kaplow, R. (2004). Applying the synergy model to nursing education. *Critical Care Nurse,* 22(Suppl. 3), 20–26.	The study linked the synergy model to the roles of a nurse educator. It used a case example to show how a nurse educator was able to use concepts from this model to educate a nurse in the critical care area.	Qualitative	Case study Level IV	**Nurse Competencies:** Clinical judgment Advocacy Caring practices Facilitation of learning Collaboration System thinking Response to diversity Clinical inquiry **Patient Characteristics:** Stability Complexity Predictability Resiliency Vulnerability Participation in decision-making Resource availability	The educator utilized patient characteristics and nursing competencies from the synergy model as strategies for intervention in the mentoring/education of the nurse. This was done to enhance patient outcomes.	Patient characteristics relate to clinical condition. The educator had more (15 years) experience compared to the nurse she was mentoring. Benner's theory, novice to expert, would have provided additional support for the insight the educator had in the clinical situation. Patient outcome was used as an evaluation of this process; however, this was not clearly stated.

Source: Scarpa, R., & Holly, C. (2010). *Systematic review of the synergy model of patient care. Proceedings of the Joanna Briggs Institute International Colloquium,* Chicago, IL.

of research results to the wider patient base, and effectiveness of the treatments. Comparisons provide a GRADE score that reflects the quality of the evidence as high, moderate, low, or very low. Quantitative findings are entered into the GRADEpro software to generate evidence profiles and summary-of- findings tables (Guyatt et al., 2008).

For qualitative reviews, CONQUAL is used to determine the level of confidence (trust) readers have in the value of the synthesized findings for informing healthcare practice and policy (Munn, Porritt, Lockwood, Aromataris, & Pearson, 2014), by assessing the dependability and credibility of the results. Dependability is laser focused on the appropriateness of the study methodology. Credibility aligns an author's explanation with the original data sources. CONQUAL determines the level of confidence for each synthesized finding and provides each finding with a score of high, moderate, low, or very low on the basis of the dependability of the primary studies from which the synthesized finding was composed and the credibility of the research findings from those studies. To assess dependability, the CONQUAL uses five questions that can be answered as "yes," "no," or "not applicable":

1. Is there congruity between the research methodology and the research question or objectives?
2. Is there congruity between the research methodology and the methods used to collect data?
3. Is there congruity between the research methodology and the representation and analysis of data?
4. Is there a statement locating the researcher culturally or theoretically?
5. Is the influence of the researcher on the research, and vice-versa, addressed?

Credibility is evaluated with the following ranking scales in the CONQUAL system: (a) unequivocal (findings accompanied by an illustration that is beyond reasonable doubt and therefore not open to challenge), (b) equivocal (findings open to challenge), (c) unsupported (findings are not supported by the data; Joanna Briggs Institute [JBI], 2014; Munn et al., 2014).

Interpret Results

When interpreting the results of a systematic review, it is important to consider the clinical relevance of the findings and whether the findings are precise enough to be used in point-of-care decision-making.

According to Burls (2009), it is imperative to determine whether there are any vital differences between the study participants and the target population that might change the effectiveness of an intervention. As Burls (2009) contends, "It is no use establishing that patients had less pain but neglecting to observe that they could be dying more often simply because this outcome was not measured" (p. 7).

The results of a systematic review of quantitative data are often reported in terms of their effect size, that is, a common metric that standardizes results across all findings, so that they can be compared. An effect size is a measure of both the strength and relationship of the variables (Lipsey & Wilson, 2001). An effect size can be any statistical test. The odds ratio (OR) is the most commonly used statistical test for determining effect size with dichotomous variables (i.e., those with only two categories: yes/no, male/female). There are several statistical tests that can be used to determine an effect size with continuous variables (i.e., those with a range of values: test scores, length of stay), including correlation coefficients and mean differences (Holly et al., 2012; Lipsey & Wilson, 2001; Littel et al., 2008). Cohen (1988) developed an often-used guide to determine whether the effect size was large, medium, or small, based on the statistical index used as follows:

- For categorical data using an odds ratio, a large effect would equal 3.4, a medium effect 2.5, and a small effect 1.5.
- For continuous data and a standard mean difference, a large effect would equal 0.8 and a small effect 0.2.

Both the Cochran Collaboration and the Joanna Briggs Institute have available software to combine findings of individual studies and produce an effect size using either an odds ratio or a standard mean difference. The results would be displayed in a forest plot (i.e., a graphic display of the results of a meta-analysis. See, for example, Holly and Slyer [2013]).

In qualitative studies, the process of meta-synthesis is used. This involves assembling findings, categorizing the findings into groups based on similarities in meaning, and aggregating these to generate a set of synthesized statements. Figure 9.2 presents this process, showing how findings are collapsed into categories and after which a synthesized statement is generated.

Report the Findings

Systematic reviews should be written according to the PRISMA (Preferred Reporting Items for Systematic Reviews and Meta-Analyses;

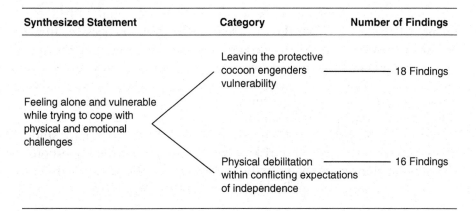

Synthesized Statement	Category	Number of Findings
Feeling alone and vulnerable while trying to cope with physical and emotional challenges	Leaving the protective cocoon engenders vulnerability	18 Findings
	Physical debilitation within conflicting expectations of independence	16 Findings

FIGURE 9.2 Findings are collapsed into categories and categories are combined into a synthesis statement.

Source: Holly, C., Salmond, S., & Saimbert, M. (2016). *Comprehensive systematic review for advanced nursing practice* (2nd ed., p. 228). New York, NY: Springer Publishing. Reprinted with permission.

www.prisma-statement.org) guidelines. The PRISMA Statement consists of a 27-item checklist and a four-phase flow diagram, and it is an expansion of the now-outdated QUOROM Statement. The checklist and flow diagram are available online in both English and Spanish. Its intent is to improve the reporting of different types of health research and in turn to improve the quality of research used in decision-making in healthcare. The broad outline of the PRISMA statement is:

- Title, which includes the words *systematic review*
- Abstract
- Introduction with review rationale and objectives
- Method with protocol description (eligibility criteria, appraisal method, search method, data elements to be collected, including summary methods, bias assessment)
- Results, including study selection, study characteristics, risk of bias results, results of individual studies, and synthesis of results
- Discussion, which includes a summary of results, limitations, and conclusions

Adapted PRISMA is a summary of the similarities and differences in objectives/purpose, methods used, and results of included reviews. Although PRISMA was originally developed for the reporting of meta-analysis, it has become the standard procedure for reporting systematic reviews of other types of healthcare research and has evolved to address both qualitative and quantitative studies in the form of adapted PRISMA. Adapted PRISMA involves the completion of a 16-item checklist. Items include questions related to the background (one question), protocol (one question), and eligibility criteria (one question); information sources (one question) and search (one question); study selection (one question); data extraction (one question); data items (one question); risk of bias in individual studies (one question); summary measures (one question); synthesis of results study (one question); study selection (one question); study characteristics (one question); risk of bias across studies (one question); and additional analyses (one question). Response options for each item are "yes," "no," and "not applicable" (Adapted PRISMA, 2016).

SYSTEMATIC REVIEW SUMMARY

Systematic reviews have been integral to the evidence-informed practice movement as a means of keeping up with the ever-increasing amount of literature on a given topic (Fineout-Overholt, O'Mathuna, & Kent, 2008). However, decision makers are increasingly faced by an abundance of such reviews. Recently, the average number of systematic reviews published each day was estimated at 11. This equates to 330 a month, or 3,960 a year (Bastian, Glasziou, & Chalmers, 2010; Li et al., 2012). Umbrella reviews (or overviews) of reviews are a logical and appropriate next step, allowing linkages to be formed from the findings of separate reviews. An umbrella review does not duplicate searches, assessment of eligibility, assessment of risk of bias, or meta-analyses from the included reviews, but it provides an overall picture of a particular phenomenon. This is a more useful and inclusive method to use to inform guidelines and clinical practice (Ionnaides, 2009).

OTHER TYPES OF REVIEWS

Rapid Reviews

Systematic reviews are complex activities, requiring substantial time and resources to meet accepted standards. Advantages include increasing statistical power, decreasing the likelihood of type II errors, minimizing the influence of bias, and transparently reporting review methods. Well-conducted systematic reviews employ high methodological standards to address healthcare questions by identifying, appraising, and summarizing primary research. A drawback of systematic reviews is that the amount of time they require to complete (6 months to up to 2 years or more) can be too long for the time-sensitive needs of decision makers. (Consider the special need for rapid advice and information during the recent Ebola epidemic.) An added constraint is that the dissemination of results is limited by the complex nature of systematic reports, which often near 100 pages. Stakeholders often require access to contextualized resources that succinctly address a broader scope of evidence in a shorter time frame than a systematic review will allow. In response, rapid reviews have emerged, allowing reviews to be completed more quickly. Schünemann and Moja (2015) maintain that rapid reviews should be conducted in less than 8 weeks. This is a time saving of about 75% compared to what most researchers identify as a standard timeline for systematic results. Other estimates for the completion of rapid review range from 5 minutes to 8 months. Consequently, a rapid review is characterized by a strong focus on the specific needs of a particular decision maker and by methodological shortcuts. These shortcuts modify the most time-consuming steps of systematic reviews, in particular, the literature search, study selection, quality assessment, and evidence synthesis. However, rapid reviews have the potential to overcome key barriers in the use of research evidence in decision-making, namely, the timely sharing of evidence. Rapid reviews allow decision makers to make decisions grounded in evidence, rather than on less robust evidence found in expert opinion or the results of a single small study. However, a rapid research search is limited to commonly used databases (often only one, such as the Cochrane Library or PubMed) and often omits dual data abstraction and critical appraisal. All of these make the validity and reliability of results questionable.

Estimates for the completion of a rapid review, alternately called *evidence summary*, ranged from 5 minutes to 8 months. Generally, rapid reviews are used to inform emergent decisions faced by decision makers in healthcare settings (Khangura, Polisena, Clifford, Farrah, & Kamel, 2014). A rapid review supplies the synthesis (qualitative and/or quantitative) needed to inform the direction and strength of the evidence.

A formal definition for a rapid review does not exist. However, a working definition provided by Khangura et al. (2014) suggests that "a rapid review is a type of knowledge synthesis in which components of the systematic review process are simplified or omitted to produce information in a short period of time" (p. 2). The following parameters are used to guide the method of a rapid review:

■ Fewer databases, often only one, are searched.

- The use of grey literature is very limited or not used at all.
- There is a restriction on the types of studies included (e.g., English only, performed with past 5 years; only systematic reviews).
- There is limited inclusion of full text; abstracts are acceptable.
- There is limited dual review for study selection and/or data extraction.
- Data extraction is limited to the basic information necessary to provide information for decision-making.
- There is limited or no grading of recommendations.
- There is limited evidence synthesis. Results are often provided as a list.
- Only minimal conclusions or recommendations are provided.

Considering the shortened time frame available for a rapid review, the methods used vary widely. As the time frames lengthen, many of the limitations can be adjusted or lifted; however, there are still restrictions on database searching, inclusion criteria, extent of data extraction, and dual review (Hartling et al., 2015).

For example, Khangura et al. (2014) describe a rapid review of the effectiveness of emergency department (ED) short-stay units. The problem under consideration was overcrowding in the ED. They used one systematic review to develop key messages for the stakeholder.

SCOPING REVIEWS

Scoping reviews are exploratory in nature. Unlike the systematic review, which uses a focused clinical question, a scoping review takes a more panoramic view. Also called *mapping reviews*, they present the literature on a topic;identify key concepts, theories, and sources of evidence; and can be used to develop working definitions, analyze concepts, or better understand a phenomenon (Peters, Godfrey, Hanan, & Baldini Soares, 2015). A scoping review is less likely to address very specific research questions or to assess the quality of included studies. Scoping reviews are often conducted before a systematic review when the achievability of research is in question, either because the relevant literature is vast and diverse (varying by methods, theoretical orientations, and disciplines) and/or because little literature exists (Colquhoun et al., 2014).

The scoping review has become an increasingly popular means of investigation by which to identify the range and nature of existing evidence and to help in the formulation of a research question(s) and the development of research proposals. Scoping reviews characteristically involve the development, assimilation, and synthesis of a broad base of evidence derived from a diverse range of research and nonresearch sources (Peters et al., 2015).

According to Arksey and O'Malley (2005), there are four common reasons to undertake a scoping review as opposed to a systematic review:

1. To map a field of study
2. To determine the feasibility of undertaking a full systematic review, including the cost of the review
3. To summarize research findings
4. To identify gaps in knowledge or research

The currently accepted method for conducting a scoping review involves steps to achieve in-depth yet broad results. All relevant literature is included without limitations on key words, type of study, or time frame. This type of review uses an iterative process, requiring researchers to reflect on each phase of the review and to repeat steps to ensure that the literature is covered in a comprehensive way (Arksey & O'Malley, 2005).

Scoping reviews can be considered a repository, useful for mapping literature and identifying when more in-depth reviews and syntheses need to be conducted. The timeliness and depth of the scoping review results are dependent on the volume of literature that exists in the particular topic area to be scoped (Brien, Lorenzetti, Lewis, Kennedy, & Ghali, 2010).

For example, in a scoping review on healthcare report cards, Brien et al. (2010) found 10,102 articles; 821 were deemed relevant to their scoping review. An additional 401 were identified from updates, website searches, references lists, review of key journals, and stakeholder suggestions, for a total of 1,222 articles included in the review.

An additional example is provided by Farebrother et al. (2015), who conducted a scoping review on iodine deficiency and its relationship to prenatal and postnatal growth in children. The scoping review was undertaken to determine the need, and to avoid duplication, for a systematic review to contribute to the evidence base in this area. Two databases were searched: TRIP (Turning Research Into Practice; www.tripdatabase.com) and Epistemonikos (www.epistemonikos.org). TRIP is a consistently updated clinical search engine focused on evidence-based medicine and clinical guidelines, including content from the Cochrane Database of Systematic Reviews (CDSR) and PubMed. Epistemonikos is an international database of research evidence that aims to provide rapid access to systematic reviews in health and that is maintained by systematically searching 25 databases for systematic reviews, broad synthesis, or structured summaries, including CDSR, PubMed, and Embase. Nine hundred and seventy-six records were screened and 10 systematic reviews were identified and included in the scoping study. Methodological quality of included reviews was assessed using AMSTAR (Assessing the Methodological Quality of Systematic Reviews). Most studies were of moderate methodological quality. This review demonstrated a gap in the evidence base with no existing up-to-date systematic reviews on the effects of all forms of iodine supplementation/fortification in the relevant population. It was concluded that a new systematic review was necessary.

REVIEWS OF TEXT AND OPINION

In the absence of qualitative or quantitative research data or when a need to support or complement existing evidence exists, a review of text and opinion is a viable option for establishing best evidence for decision-making. An important consideration in the decision to use text and opinion as evidence is to be transparent when opinion is the evidence being used so that practitioners and decision makers can make independent decisions as to the validity of the recommendations based on the opinion (Woolf, 2000). McArthur, Klugarova, Yan, & Florescu (2015) also suggest that the opinion of one expert is not as valid as the consensus of a group of experts and this needs to be taken into consideration when reviewing the opinion-based recommendations. Although it is important to recognize that text and opinion may not be the high-quality evidence associated with a systematic review, it is possible that no research exists on a given topic, as many clinical practices are based on practitioners' tacit knowledge, experience, or current discussion within a community of interest. Text and opinion can combine the collective wisdom of practitioners to provide practical guidance (Jordan, Konno, & Mu, 2011; McArthur et al., 2015). This narrative expression of clinical wisdom and insight may not easily be reconciled with inductive and deductive reasoning (McArthur et al., 2015; Worth, 2008). Text and opinion can be derived from:

- Consensus reports and guidelines
- Expert opinion
- Monographs
- White papers bt professional organizations
- Nonresearch-based journal articles
- Standards of care
- Conference proceedings

- Policy reports
- Industry-based technical reports (e.g., pharmaceutical or medical device industry)

In addition to the major databases, such as Medline, Embase, or CINAHL, searching the grey literature is important to identifying text and opinion narratives and, in some instances, may provide the primary source for identification of relevant opinion. As reviews of text and opinion are not based on traditional research, the words *text* or *narrative* should be included in the search terms, rather than *study*.

CONCLUSIONS

A systematic review provides a high level of evidence on the effectiveness of healthcare interventions and the nuances of observation that can be used to inform recommendations for practice. These reviews are complex and largely dependent upon finding the best evidence. However, a systematic review can advise what is known, what is not known, and what needs to be known about a specific clinical topic.

■ QUESTIONS FOR DISCUSSION

1. What is the value of doing a systematic review for doctor of nursing practice (DNP)?
2. Should the method of systematic review be included in all DNP programs of study?

■ REFLECTIVE EXERCISE

Read the following systematic review. Determine how the critical appraisal process was conducted. Write a letter to the editor regarding the adequacy of the appraisal process.

Holly, C., Porter, S., Echevarria, M., Drecker, M., & Ruzhaji, S. (2018). Recognizing delirium in hospitalized children: A systematic review of risk factors and characteristics of acute pediatric delirium. *American Journal of Nursing, 118*(4), 24–26. doi:10.1097/01. NAJ.0000532069.55339.f9

EXAMPLES OF SYSTEMATIC REVIEWS

Recognizing Delirium in Hospitalized Children: A Systematic Review of Risk Factors and Characteristics of Acute Pediatric Delirium

The purpose of this review was to examine the evidence on risk factors and characteristics of acute pediatric delirium. Using the systematic review method within an epidemiological framework of person, time, and place, a total of 52 studies were selected for retrieval and 21 (N=2616) were included after assessment for methodological quality using tools validated for this purpose. Findings reveal that there are five primary characteristics seen in children experiencing delirium: inattention, agitation, sleep–wake cycle disturbances, impaired orientation, and hallucinations, usually visual. Children who were more seriously ill, such as those in the pediatric intensive care unit (PICU) with a high pediatric risk of mortality II (PRISM II) score orchildren who were mechanically ventilated, were at greater risk for developing delirium. Those with a developmental delay or a preexisting anxiety disorder were also more prone to delirium. Although delirium symptoms fluctuate, most episodes occurred at night. Delirium is multifactorial. It is related to treatment (e.g., mechanical ventilation) and the hospital environment (PICU) and deprives patients of normal sleep–wake cycles and familiar routines. Early recognition and management of pediatric delirium may help prevent unnecessary laboratory testing and imaging studies that increase overall hospital cost as well as inflict unnecessary pain and anxiety on children.

Source: Holly, C., Porter, S., Echevarria, M., Drecker, M., & Ruzhaji, S. (2018). Recognizing delirium in hospitalized children: A systematic review of risk factors and characteristics of acute pediatric delirium. *American Journal of Nursing, 118*(4), 24–26. doi:10.1097/01.NAJ.0000532069.55339.f9

A Systematic Review of the Effectiveness of Three Methods of Fentanyl Administration Following Discharge From Acute Care

The aim of this systematic review was to examine the evidence on the effectiveness of fentanyl modalities for the adult cancer patient. Modes of administration reviewed were transdermal, buccal, intranasal, and oral transmucosal. A secondary aim of the review is to describe cost utility and cost effectiveness between various modes of fentanyl administration.

The search strategy aimed to find both published and unpublished studies. A four-step search strategy was utilized in this review. First, a limited search of Medline and CINAHL was undertaken using the key words *fentanyl, adult cancer patient,* and *chronic pain management.* This was followed by analysis of the text words contained in the title and abstract of all identified papers. A second search using the expanded list was then undertaken across all included databases. Third, the reference list of all articles was searched for additional studies. Studies published in the English language and available in full text were considered for inclusion in this review. Finally, five journals specific to the topic were hand searched. These included *AANA Journal, Pain and Analgesia Journal, Journal of Pharmacology, Nurse Economics,* and *Cancer Nursing.* Two reviewers independently assessed all studies identified from the search strategy against

(continued)

EXAMPLES OF SYSTEMATIC REVIEWS (*CONTINUED*)

the inclusion criteria. In the third step, studies that met the inclusion criteria were further assessed for methodological quality using standardized critical appraisal instruments. More than 700 potential studies were identified. Of these, 16 studies were retrieved for appraisal and 11 included in this review: nine randomized controlled trials on the effectiveness of fentanyl and two on the economics of fentanyl use (one cost-utility study and one cost-effectiveness study). Due to heterogeneity, a meta-analysis was not possible, and studies were presented as a narrative. The findings of this review suggest that fentanyl provides adequate pain relief alone and may be more effective than other methods studied, such as tramadol, methadone, Dilaudid, or morphine, in relieving pain in the adult cancer patient. Fentanyl in spray form had a more rapid onset than other drugs used for breakthrough pain (level 1). Fentanyl was found to be cost-effective and increased quality of life (level 2).

Source: Guilante, M. A., Antonio, A., & Duncan, K. (2011). *A systematic review of the effectiveness of three methods of fentanyl administration following discharge from acute care.* In C. Holly (Ed.), *Scholarly inquiry and the DNP capstone.* New York, NY: Springer Publishing.

■ SUGGESTED READINGS

Deeks, J. J. (2001). Systematic reviews of evaluation of diagnostic and screening tests. In M. Egger, G. D. Smith, & G. D. Altman (Eds.), *Systematic review in healthcare: Meta-analysis in context* (2nd ed., pp. 248–280). London, England: BMJ.

Hanes, K., Lockwood, C., & Pearson, A. (2010). A comparative analysis of three appraisal instruments to assess validity in qualitative research. *Qualitative Health Research, 20*(12), 1736–1743. doi:10.1177/1049732310378656

Higgins, J. P. T., & Thompson, S. G. (2002). Quantifying heterogeneity in a meta-analysis. *Statistics in Medicine, 21,* 1539–1558. doi:10.1002/sim.1186

Moher, D., Liberati, A., Tetzlaff, J., Altman, D. G., & PRISMA Group. (2009). Preferred reporting items for systematic reviews and meta-analyses: The PRISMA statement. *PLoS Medicine, 6*(7), e1000097. doi:10.1371/journal.pmed.1000097

■ REFERENCES

Adapted PRISMA. (2016). Retrieved from http://cjasn.asnjournals.org/site/misc/Prisma Checklist.pdf

Arksey, H., & O'Malley, L. (2005). Scoping studies: Towards a methodological framework. *International Journal of Social Research Methodology, 8*(1), 19–32.

Bahekar, A. A., Singh, S., Saha, S., Molnar, J., & Arora, R. (2007). The prevalence and incidence of coronary heart disease is significantly increased in periodontitis: A meta-analysis. *American Heart Journal, 154*(5), 830–837.

Bastian, H., Glasziou, P., & Chalmers, I. (2010). Seventy-five trials and eleven systematic reviews a day: How will we ever keep up? *PLoS Medicine, 7*(9), e1000326. doi:10.1371/journal.pmed.1000326

Brien, S., Lorenzetti, D., Lewis, S., Kennedy, J., & Ghali, W. (2010). Overview of a formal scoping review on health system report cards. *Implementation Science, 5*, 2–10.

Burls, A. (2009). *What is critical appraisal?* London, England: Hayworth Press.

Chalmers, I. (2006). *The scandalous failure of scientists to cumulate scientifically.* Abstract to paper presented at: Ninth World Congress on Health Information and Libraries, Salvador, Brazil. Retrieved from www.icml9.org/program/public/documents/Chalmers-131528.pdf

Childress, S. (2013). A meta-summary of qualitative findings on the lived experience among culturally diverse domestic violence survivors. *Issues in Mental Health Nursing, 34*(9), 693–705. doi:10.3109/01612840.2013.791735

Cohen, J. (1988). *Statistical power analysis for the behavioral sciences.* New York, NY: Academic Press.

Colquhoun, H. L., Levac, D., O'Brien, K. K., Straus, S., Tricco, A. C., Perrier, L., . . . Moher, D. (2014). Scoping reviews: Time for clarity in definition, methods, and reporting. *Journal of Clinical Epidemiology, 67*(12), 1291–1294.

Doi, S. A., & Thalib, L. (2008). A quality-effects model for meta-analysis. *Epidemiology, 19*(1), 94–100. doi:10.1097/EDE.0b013e31815c24e7

Farebrother, J., Naude, C. E., Nicol, L., Sang, Z., Yang, Z., Andersson, M., . . . Zimmermann, M. B. (2015). Systematic review of the effects of iodised salt and iodine supplements on prenatal and postnatal growth: Study protocol. *BMJ Open, 5*(4), e007238.

Fineout-Overholt, E., O'Mathuna, D. P., & Kent, B. (2008). How systematic reviews can foster evidence-based clinical decisions. *Worldviews on Evidence-Based Nursing, 5*, 45–48. doi:10.1111/j.1741-6787.2008.00116.x

Glass, G. V. (1978). Primary, secondary, and meta-analysis of research. *Educational Researcher, 5*(10), 3–8. doi:10.3102/0013189X005010003

Guilante, M. A., Antonio, A., & Duncan, K. (2011). *A systematic review of the effectiveness of three methods of fentanyl administration following discharge from acute care.* In C. Holly (Ed.), *Scholarly inquiry and the DNP capstone.* New York, NY: Springer Publishing.

Guyatt, G. H., Oxman, A. D., Vist, G. E., Kunz, R., Falck-Ytter, Y., Alonso-Coello, P., & Schünemann, H. J. (2008). GRADE: An emerging consensus on rating quality of evidence and strength of recommendations. *BMJ, 336*, 924. doi:10.1136/bmj.39489.470347.AD

Hartling, L., Guise, J. M., Kato, E., Anderson, J., Belinson, S., Berliner, E., . . . Whitlock, E. (2015). A taxonomy of rapid reviews links report types and methods to specific decision-making contexts. *Journal of Clinical Epidemiology, 68*(12), 1451–1462.e3.

Higgins, J. P. T., & Thompson, S. G. (2002). Quantifying heterogeneity in a meta-analysis. *Statistics in Medicine, 21*, 1539–1558. doi:10.1002/sim.1186

Higgins, J. P. T., Thompson, S. G., Deeks, J. J., & Altman, D. G. (2003). Measuring inconsistency in meta-analyses. *British Medical Journal, 327*, 557–560. doi:10.1136/bmj.327.7414.557

Ho, K. H., & Chiang, V. C. (2015). A meta-ethnography of the acculturation and socialization experiences of migrant care workers. *Journal of Advanced Nursing, 71*(2), 237–254. doi:10.1111/jan.12506

Holly, C., Porter, S., Echevarria, M., Drecker, M., & Ruzhaji, S. (2018). Recognizing delirium in hospitalized children: A systematic review of risk factors and characteristics of acute pediatric delirium. *American Journal of Nursing, 118*(4), 24–26. doi:10.1097/01.NAJ.0000532069.55339.f9

Holly, C., Salmond, S., & Saimbert, M. (2012). *Comprehensive systematic review for advanced nursing practice.* New York, NY: Springer Publishing.

Holly, C., Salmond, S., & Saimbert, M. (2016). *Comprehensive systematic review for advanced nursing practice* (2nd ed.). New York, NY: Springer Publishing.

Holly, C., & Slyer, J. (2013). Interpreting and using meta-analysis in clinical practice. *Orthopedic Nursing, 32*(2), 106–110. doi:10.1097/NOR.0b013e3182879c34

Ionnaides, J. (2009). Integration of evidence from multiple meta-analyses: a primer on umbrella reviews, treatment networks and multiple treatments meta-analyses. *CMAJ, 181*(8), 488–493. doi:10.1503/cmaj.081086

Joanna Briggs Institute. (2014). *Joanna Briggs Institute reviewers' manual 2014*. Adelaide, AU: University of Adelaide.

Jordan, Z., Konno, R., & Mu, P. F. (2011). *Synthesizing evidence from narrative, text and opinion*. Philadelphia, PA: Lippincott Williams & Wilkins.

Kaplow, R. (2004). Applying the synergy model to nursing education. *Critical Care Nurse, 22*(Suppl. 3), 20–26.

Khangura, S., Polisena, J., Clifford, T. J., Farrah, K., & Kamel, C. (2014). Rapid review: An emerging approach to evidence synthesis in health technology assessment. *International Journal of Technology Assessment in Health Care, 30*(1), 20–27.

Kitchenham, B. (2004). *Procedures for systematic review: Joint technical report*. Retrieved from http://csnotes.upm.edu.my/kelasmaya/pgkm20910.nsf/0/715071a8011d4c2f482577a700386d3a/$FILE/10.1.1.122.3308%5B1%5D.pdf

Li, L., Tian, J., Tian, H., Sun, R., Liu, Y., & Yang, K. (2012). Quality and transparency of overviews of systematic reviews. *JEBM, 5*, 166–173. doi:10.1111/j.1756-5391.2012.01185.x

Lipsey, M., & Wilson, D. (2001). *Practical meta-analysis*. Thousand Oaks, CA: Sage.

Littell, J. H., Corcoran, J., & Pillai, V. (2008). *Systematic reviews and meta-analysis*. Oxford, UK: Oxford University Press.

McArthur, A., Klugarova, J., Yan, H., & Florescu, S. (2015). Innovations in the systematic review of text and opinion. *International Journal of Evidence-Based Healthcare, 13*(3), 188–195.

MetaXL. (2012). Retrieved from http://www.epigear.com/index_files/metaxl.html

Munn, Z., Porritt, K., Lockwood, C., Aromataris, E., & Pearson, A. (2014). Establishing confidence in the output of qualitative research synthesis: The ConQual approach. *BMC Medical Research Methodology 14*(1), 108. doi:10.1186/1471-2288-14-108

Peters, M., Godfrey, C. M., Hanan, K., & Baldini Soares, C. (2015). Guidance for conducting systematic scoping reviews. *International Journal of Evidence-Based Healthcare, 13*(3), 141–146.

Scarpa, R., & Holly, C. (2010). *Systematic review of the synergy model of patient care*. Proceedings of the Joanna Briggs Institute International Colloquium, Chicago, IL.

Schünemann, H. J., & Moja, L. (2015). Reviews: Rapid! Rapid! Rapid! . . . and systematic. *Systematic Reviews, 14*(4), 4.

Vaismoradi, M., Skär, L., Söderberg, S., & Bondas, T. E. (2016). Normalizing suffering: A meta-synthesis of experiences of and perspectives on pain and pain management in nursing homes. *International Journal of Qualitative Studies on Health and Well-Being, 11*, 31203. doi:10.3402/qhw.v11.31203

Woolf, S. H. (2000). Evidence-based medicine and practice guide-lines: An overview. *Cancer Control, 7*, 362–367.

Worth, S. E. (2008). Storytelling and narrative knowing: An examination of the epistemic benefits of well-told stories. *Journal of Aesthetic Education, 42*(3), 42–56.

CHAPTER 10

Integrative Review

■ OBJECTIVES

At the end of this chapter, you will be able to:

- Differentiate between a review of the literature, an integrative review, and a systematic review.
- Determine which of the review types will best answer your question.
- Describe the steps needed to conduct an integrative review of the literature.

■ KEY CONCEPTS

- An integrative review of the literature is a summary of literature on a particular topic.
- Rigorous integrative reviews can contribute to theory development.
- Integrative reviews are useful for keeping current with the ever-expanding volume of literature.
- Integrative reviews summarize what is known at a particular point in time.
- An integrative review of the literature has a broader focus than a traditional review of the literature, but not the focused clinical question associated with a systematic review.

INTRODUCTION

Integrative reviews instill nursing practice with evidence to provide solutions to clinical problems. An integrative review is not a research

© Springer Publishing Company DOI: 10.1891/9780826134943.0010   171

method, nor can an integrative review of the literature review be used as a synonym for a literature review, systematic review, or meta-analysis. See Table 10.1 for a comparison of these review methods. An integrative literature review summarizes the main points of past research to draw general conclusions from a literary source on a certain topic using literature that includes studies that address related or identical hypotheses (https://guides.temple.edu/c.php?g=78618&p=4260131). Essentially, it is a critical summary of literature on a particular topic. As such, an integrative review appraises and combines available evidence, including theory. The integrative review method can incorporate diverse methodologies to capture the circumstances, processes, and individual elements of the topic under study (Whittemore & Knafl, 2005). It takes a traditional review of the literature one step further by providing a more substantial contribution to knowledge using a transparent process. It may also involve a critical appraisal of the literature used in the review. New perspectives and frameworks can be generated through an integrative review, and research questions can be developed for further study. An integrative review of the literature has a broader focus than a traditional review of the literature, but not the focused clinical question

TABLE 10.1

TYPES OF REVIEW

	Literature Review	Integrative Review	Systematic Review
Focus	Broad	Defined	Precise
Search strategy	Limited to material that is 5 years old; may include a search of only one database or search engine	Search is based on key words; pivotal papers are searched for in three to six databases or search engines	An exhaustive search, including hand searching and a search for unpublished (gray) literature; uses an explicit strategy
Appraisal	Appraisal is done to establish support for the research question	Appraisal may be rigorous but may be done by only one reviewer	Rigorous appraisal by two independent reviewers; uses valid and reliable tools for appraisal based on the study's research design
Outcome	Background	Recommendations	Best practice

associated with a systematic review. There are many benefits to an integrative review, including:

- Definition of concepts
- Review and comparison of theories
- Analysis of methodological issues on a particular topic
- Accentuation of unresolved issues or gaps in knowledge
- Identification of trends
- Evaluation of current practices

Conducting an integrative literature review involves the same rigor used when conducting primary research. At first, there are four questions to ask when considering an integrative review of the literature (Russell, 2005):

- What is known?
- What is the quality of what is known?
- What should be known?
- What is the next step for research or practice?

STEPS IN AN INTEGRATIVE REVIEW

Step One: Selecting the Question for Review

The task of developing guiding questions to focus the review is of immense importance. These questions provide direction for all other phases of the review. The questions should flow from the aim or purpose of the review. See Box 10.1 for an example. Key concepts, such as the population for study, any interventions of interest, comparison groups, and outcomes, should be evident in the guiding questions. Well-stated guiding questions will help to resolve any ambiguity in the review and facilitate in delineating the scope of the review (Broome, 2000).

The scope, or range, of the review is of importance. If a number of studies have been conducted on the question of interest, the reviewer needs to narrow the question. On the other hand, if the topic has little research available, the question may need to be expanded. Russell (2005) provides this example:

If the reviewer's initial research question is "What interventions are most effective in increasing treatment compliance in liver transplant recipients?" but no intervention studies have been conducted with this population, then the reviewer may need to

BOX 10.1

EXAMPLE OF GUIDING QUESTIONS FOR AN INTEGRATIVE REVIEW

The objective of this integrative review was to examine the evidence on factors that influence and strategies that support the academic success of culturally diverse students. Specifically, the questions that guided the review were:

1. What are the facilitators and barriers to successful completion of a nursing program for culturally diverse students?
2. What are the strategies that support success in the NCLEX-RN® (National Council Licensure Examination) exam for culturally diverse students?
3. What are the characteristics of successful retention programs for culturally diverse students?

Source: Cantwell, E. R., & Holly, C. (2012). *An integrative review on the best strategies to assist culturally diverse nursing students toward successful program completion.* Unpublished manuscript. Retrieved from hollych@umdnj.edu

broaden the research question to, "What interventions are the most effective in increasing treatment compliance in all transplant recipients?" (p. 2)

Guiding questions for an integrative review are background questions. Background questions ask for general knowledge about an illness, disease, condition, process, or concept. These types of questions typically ask who, what, where, when, how, and why about a disorder, test, or treatment. Guiding questions used should clearly delineate the key words and phrases needed to search the literature. For example:

■ What are the clinical manifestations of delirium?
■ What are the experiences nursing staff regarding family-witnessed resuscitation?
■ How is resilience manifested in the pediatric population?
■ What are some common indications for a transesophageal echocardiogram?
■ When do complications of elective hysterectomy usually occur?
■ What are common characteristics of patients exhibiting drug-seeking behavior?

Step Two: Locating the Right Studies for Inclusion in the Review

The search for the right studies to include in the integrative review occurs during the data-collection phase. Using the key words and phrases garnered from the guiding questions, a search strategy is developed. The search should be broad and encompass a minimum of two databases, although a search of three to six databases is preferred. This search of databases is different from a systematic review, in which as many databases as necessary are searched so that the search is exhaustive. The strategy developed should include an electronic database search, a hand search in journals relevant to the guiding questions, and a search of the reference list of studies selected to be included in the review. A search for gray or unpublished literature can be considered, but it is not necessary. Authors who have previously published on the topic for review can be contacted to determine whether any other sources are available or if they have published similar papers. At the end of the search, the reviewer should have in hand all of the evidence that could potentially be used in the review.

Some of the common databases that can be searched for an integrative review on a nursing topic include:

1. Academic Search Premier, which contains indexing and abstracts for more than 8,500 journals, with full text for more than 4,600 of those titles related to health, medicine, and biology, among others. It also contains authors' contact information, which can be useful in identifying other relevant studies for inclusion in the review.

2. Medline (Medical Literature Analysis and Retrieval System Online) is a database of life sciences and biomedical information compiled by the National Library of Medicine. It includes information for articles from academic journals covering medicine, nursing, pharmacy, dentistry, veterinary medicine, and healthcare. PubMed is the search engine used to access Medline.

3. CINAHL (Cumulative Index of Nursing and Allied Health Literature) is a database of nursing and allied health literature with indexing of more than 3,000 journals and more than 2.6 million records dating back to 1981. In addition, this database offers access to healthcare books, nursing dissertations, selected conference proceedings, standards of practice, educational software, audiovisuals, and book chapters.

4. Web of Science, which is an online academic citation index provided by Thomson Reuters. It allows access to multiple databases for cross-disciplinary research and in-depth exploration of specialized subfields within an academic or scientific discipline. As a citation index, any cited paper will lead to other literature (book, academic journal, proceedings, etc.) that has currently, or in the past, cited this work.
5. Mednaris a free, publicly available search engine that does deep web searches. It includes a search of the Cochrane Library, Google Scholar, PubMed/Medline, and all National Institutes of Health (NIH) websites.

The search should look for primary, secondary, and tertiary literature. *Primary literature* refers to an original study, or primary research. Primary literature is an original work or firsthand account describing a phenomenon or experiment. For example, Hartog et al. (2010) studied the neurological outcomes of patients admitted to an ICU with temperatures below 95°F. Secondary literature summarizes and synthesizes primary literature. Secondary literature includes meta-analyses, metasyntheses, and systematic reviews. Textbooks are also considered a type of secondary literature. Completed secondary literature reports on medical, nursing, and other health profession literature can be found in the Cochrane Library (www.cochrane.org) or the Joanna Briggs Library (www.joannabrigg.edu.au). The Campbell Collaborative houses completed systematic reviews on educational, psychological, and social topics, including criminal justice (www.campbellcollaboration.org). Tertiary literature includes a summary or an abstract of primary or secondary literature. Online databases, such as WebMD (www.webmd.com) or Dynamed (dynamed.ebscohost.com), are tertiary literature sites (Holly, Salmond, & Saimbert, 2016).

A best practice for conducting literature searches is to search one electronic resource at a time. Searching multiple databases at once should be avoided. Each database has specific features that will not be the same as those in another database, so some article citations may be missed. Searching across databases is known as *federated* or *cross-database* searching. An example of a federated search includes clicking a button in Ovid to search Medline and Books@Ovid and the PsycINFO databases all at once (Holly et al.,2016).

For example, in an integrative review of postcraniotomy pain in the patient with a brain tumor, Guilkey, Von Ah, Carpenter, Stone, and Draucker (2016) identified relevant literature using the key words *traumatic brain injury, pain, postoperative, brain injuries, postoperative pain, craniotomy, decompressive craniectomy,* and *trephining.* They searched Medline, Ovid, PubMed, and CINAHL databases from 2000 to 2014. The search yielded 115 manuscripts, with 26 meeting inclusion criteria. Most studies were randomized controlled trials conducted outside of the United States. All tested pharmacological pain interventions.

Step Three: Representing the Findings of the Studies

To assist in having a review that contains only the best available evidence, each of the selected studies needs to be critically appraised. Holly et al. (2016) have noted that "the critical appraisal provides a balanced assessment of the benefits and strengths of the research against its flaws and weaknesses" (p. 148). The focus in a critical appraisal is on the validity, reliability, and rigor of the study. Studies not meeting the appraisal criteria are excluded. *Validity* refers to the legitimacy of the findings, in other words, how authentic, truthful, and accurate they are. *Reliability* refers to the consistency of the findings, and *rigor* refers to the exactness with which the research study was designed. To determine how valid, reliable, and rigorous a study is, papers need to be read several times when doing a critical appraisal. Greenhalgh (2014) reminds us that the goal of critical appraisal is not finding methodologically flawless papers, that in reality there are flaws in 99% of all research studies. Rather, the aim is to identify papers that are *good enough.* In other words, those papers with the indicators deemed to show quality can be considered good enough.

Critical appraisal for an integrative review can be completed by one investigator. In comparison, a critical appraisal for a systematic review must be completed by two reviewers working independently. A review of the literature generally does not undergo a critical appraisal.

A detailed log of the papers determined not to be good enough for inclusion should be kept and the reason for exclusion noted.

An appraisal focuses on the adequacy of reporting data-collection methods, appropriate data analysis, and whether key findings were reported appropriately. Questions to ask when determining whether a study is appropriate for an integrative review include:

- Is the study question relevant to my guiding questions and target population?

- Does the study add anything new or support current thinking or theory on the topic?
- Was the study design appropriate for the research question?
- Did the study methods address the most important potential sources of bias? These can include selection bias (a differential selection of subjects for comparison groups), attrition (loss of subjects to follow-up), or instrumentation (changes in calibration of a measurement tool or changes in the observers or scorers that can produce changes in the outcome measured).
- Was the appropriate analytic method chosen and was it performed correctly?
- Are the conclusions based on the data?

Alternately, a critical appraisal tool, such as those developed by the Critical Skills Appraisal Programme (CASP), can be used. These appraisal tools are based upon the research study design and can be accessed for free (www.casp-uk.net/).

When the critical appraisal has been completed, a table can be created that contains information about each of the studies in the review. Called a *table of inclusion*, it should contain information about:

- The author, title, and source of the paper
- Purpose of the study
- Study design
- Sample size and major characteristics
- How the data were collected and analyzed
- Major findings
- Comments

Step Four: Analyzing the Findings

The findings of studies that have been appraised and are to be used in the study need to be extracted. To guarantee relevancy and accuracy when extracting data from a selected study, a tool should be used. Extracted data should include definition of the subjects, methodology, size of the sample, variables, method of analysis, and results. Categories and data-display matrices are then developed to display all of the data from each study by its category.

Next, these categories are compared further. As data are conceptualized at higher and higher levels of abstraction, each primary source is reread and reviewed to verify that the new conceptualization was congruent with primary sources. The overall process involves data reduction, data display, data comparison, drawing conclusion, and verification (Whittemore & Knafl, 2005).

Cooper (1998) in an old, but still relevant publication, reminds us that this step reduces individual data points for aggregation of findings. Statistical tests may or may not be used. For example, if an understanding of the concept of interprofessional collaboration is the goal of the review, statistical analysis is not necessary. On the other hand, if a review of the predictors or collaboration was the focus of the integrative review, some statistical testing may be appropriate.

Step Five: Summarizing Results

Drawing conclusions and summarizing results is the final step in an integrative review, and it is generally done as a narrative. Similarities and differences in the findings are identified and a description of generalizations representative of the defined categories are provided (Whittemore & Knafl, 2005). Findings can be presented as a research agenda that poses new questions for investigation or a taxonomy that can be used to classify previous research.

REPORTING THE INTEGRATIVE REVIEW

There is no one standard template for reporting integrative research reviews. A suggested format is to follow the general outline used for primary research, which includes Introduction, Methods, Results, and Discussion sections (Box 10.2). This should be a fully synthesized report showing the themes that emerged across the included studies. The introduction should include the list of guiding questions developed for the review and definitions of the conceptual and operational variables that were a part of the review. The Methods section should be transparent in its description of the search strategy used to locate the papers included in the review. An example of the search strategy should be included in a table or in an appendix. The approach to analyzing the data and generating themes or categories should be described. The Results section should summarize and synthesize the themes that were uncovered in the review. Finally, in the Discussion section, inferences should be drawn and discussed in relation to the guiding questions.

BOX 10.2

THE INTEGRATIVE REVIEW REPORT

Introduction
State the problems, purpose, and significance of the topic.
Describe the population to be studied.
Describe the variables under study.
State the method used for organizing the data.
List the question(s) that focus the review.

Method
Specify the search strategy.
Describe methods for identifying, obtaining, and including studies in the review.
State the databases searched.
Describe any appraisal methods used and the results.
Describe the method used to synthesize the data.

Results
Present results of data analysis.
Develop conclusions.

Discussion
Present common themes.
Discuss the results in terms of the original questions identified.
Draw inferences from the results of the synthesis.
Identify limitations of the review.

References
List all references cited in the report.

CONCLUSIONS

The integrative literature review has many benefits to a scholarly inquiry, including identifying gaps in current research, evaluating the strength of available research, and providing a strong foundation for primary research studies. Although it is not a research method, an integrative review can provide important information for conductingprimary or translational studies.

■ QUESTIONS FOR DISCUSSION

1. What has been your experience when searching for information on a clinical topic?

2. Do you think the critical appraisal step is necessary in an integrative review?
3. All of the steps in an integrative review can be done by one person. Do you think that there is any bias in this approach?

■ REFLECTIVE EXERCISE

When discharged patients transition from the acute care settings back to their community, follow-up by home healthcare nurses may be necessary

EXAMPLES OF INTEGRATIVE REVIEWS

Mentoring in Nursing: An Integrative Review of Commentaries, Editorials, and Perspectives Papers

To address the gap in knowledge about the mentoring relationship and circumnavigate mentoring's context-specific nature, this review analyzed the perspectives and opinions of nurse mentors and mentees. The purpose of the review was to identify common themes in their mentoring experiences to better nurture effective mentoring relationships and programs in nursing using editorials and perspective, reflective, narrative, and opinion pieces, which are an untapped source of information that offer insight into the long-term effects of mentoring on clinical practice, behavior of mentors and mentees, and factors that they believe are instrumental to their mentoring experiences. Thematic analysis of 35 included papers revealed five themes. These themes were common features of mentoring among featured descriptions and definitions, mentoring relationships, mentor-related aspects, host organization-related aspects, and mentee-related aspects.

Reference

Lin, J., Chew, Y. R., Toh, Y. P., & Radha-Krishna, L. K. (2018). Mentoring in nursing: An integrative review of commentaries, editorials, and perspectives papers. *Nurse Educator, 43*(1), E1–E5. doi:10.1097/NNE.0000000000000389

An Integrative Review as the Foundation for Development of a Medication Safety Program for Undergraduate Nursing Students

The purpose of the project was to conduct an integrative review of the literature related to medication communication; medication safety; and the use of the situation, background, assessment, recommendation (SBAR) technique in an acute care context and to design a medication safety program focusing on improving communication. The integrative review followed a five-step evidence-based process that included the following: Step1: problem identification, wherein the review was guided by questions developed using the population, intervention, comparison, outcomes (PICO) approach; step 2: literature search, wherein key words were used to acquire evidence via an electronic search, a hand search, and the search of reference lists; step 3: data appraisal, wherein a valid and reliable appraisal tool was used

(*continued*)

EXAMPLES OF INTEGRATIVE REVIEWS (*CONTINUED*)

for verification of methodological quality; step 4: data extraction, wherein the appraised evidence was applied to the project via the use of a table of evidence that was used as a data-extraction tool that included the source, study purpose, study design, discussion, and level of evidence; and step 5: implement and evaluate, wherein the lesson plan was developed as per the evidence and reviewed by an expert review panel that included nursing faculty who taught pharmacology and nursing faculty with a background in risk management.

The initial search found 350 relevant articles. After a review of the title and abstract, 77 were retrieved for appraisal and 31 were included in this review. Three themes were generated through the integrative review: (a) improving medication safety involves attention to communication and team relationships, (b) the use of SBAR increases students' confidence and willingness to report to colleagues, (c) enhanced communication skills reduce medication errors. The findings of the integrative review were used to develop a plan for a medication safety program titled, "Communication Is Key: Using SBAR for Medication Safety." The program was reviewed by an expert panel of doctor of nursing practice and PhD nursing faculty for feasibility and applicability, who provided recommendations for improvement.

Reference

Biddle, J. (2011). An integrative review as the foundation for development of a medication safety program for undergraduate nursing students. In, C. Holly (Ed.), *Scholarly inquiry and the DNP capstone*. New York, NY: Springer Publishing.

to prevent readmission. Write the guiding question for an integrative review of heart failure patients who are transitioning back to the community and are being followed by a home healthcare nurse. What would the nurse need to know and what follow-up strategies would she or he use? Then devise a search strategy to find papers relevant to this topic.

■ SUGGESTED READINGS

Buccheri, R., & Sharifi, C. (2017). Critical appraisal tools and reporting guidelines for evidence-based practice. *Worldviews on Evidence-Based Nursing, 14*(6), 463–472. doi:10.1111/wvn.12258

Google. (2015). Google search help. How to search on Google. Retrieved from https://support.google.com/websearch/answer/134479?hl=en&ref_topic=3081620&vid=0-635802591522179323-4179845653

McGowan, J., Sampson, M., & Lefebvre, C. (2010). An evidence based checklist for the peer review of electronic search strategies (PRESS EBC). *Evidence Based Library and*

Information Practice, 5(1), 149–154. Retrieved from http://ejournals.library.ualberta.ca
/index.php/EBLIP/article/view/7402/6436
Whittemore, R., & Knafl K. (2005). The integrative review: Updated methodology. *Journal of Advanced Nursing,* 52(5), 546–553. doi:10.1111/j.1365-2648.2005.03621.x

■ REFERENCES

Biddle, J. (2011). An integrative review as the foundation for development of a medication safety program for undergraduate nursing students. In C. Holly (Ed.), *Scholarly inquiry and the DNP capstone.* New York, NY: Springer Publishing.

Broome, M. E. (2000). Integrative literature reviews for the development of concepts. In B. Rogers& K. Knafl (Eds.), *Concept development in nursing* (pp. 231–250). Philadelphia, PA: W. B. Saunders.

Cooper, H. M. (1998). *Synthesizing research: A guide for literature reviews* (3rd ed.). Thousand Oaks, CA: Sage.

Greenhalgh, T. (2014). *How to read a paper.* London, UK: Wiley/Blackwell.

Guilkey, R. E., Von Ah, D., Carpenter, J. S., Stone, C., & Draucker, C. B. (2016). Integrative review: Postcraniotomy pain in the brain tumour patient. *Journal of Advanced Nursing,* 72(6), 1221–1235. doi:10.1111/jan.12890

Hartog, A., dePont, A., Robillard, L., Binnekade, J., Schultz, M., & Horn, J (2010). Spontaneous hypothermia on intensive care unit admission is a predictor of unfavorable neurological outcome in patients after resuscitation: An observational cohort study. *Critical Care, 14,* R121. doi:10.1186/cc9077

Holly, C., Salmond, S., & Saimbert, M. (2016). *Comprehensive systematic review for advanced nursing practice* (2nd ed.). New York, NY: Springer Publishing.

Russell, C. L. (2005). An overview of the integrative research review. *Progress in Transplantation, 15*(1), 8–13. Retrieved from http://www.nitiphong.com/paper_pdf/phd/An%20overview%20of%20the%20integrative%20research%20review.pdf

Torraco, R. J. (2005). Writing integrative literature reviews: Guidelines and examples. *Human Resource Development Review, 4,* 356. Retrieved from http://hrd.sagepub.com/content/4/3/356

Whittemore, R., & Knafl, K. (2005). The integrative review: Updated methodology. *Journal of Advanced Nursing,* 52(5), 546–553. doi:10.1111/j.1365-2648.2005.03621.x

CHAPTER 11

Quality Improvement

■ OBJECTIVES

At the end of this chapter, you will be able to:

- Define *quality improvement*.
- Differentiate between quality-improvement studies and research studies.
- Select a method for a quality-improvement study.
- Determine the appropriate quality-management tool to use to assess outcomes.
- Describe the Centers for Medicare & Medicaid Services (CMS) initiative on Meaningful Measures.

■ KEY CONCEPTS

- *Quality* implies use of a continuous monitoring process.
- Quality improvement is a focus on the structure, process, and outcomes of healthcare.
- Quality improvement has its own validated methods and tools for analysis.
- Efforts to improve quality need to be measured.

INTRODUCTION

Quality is an abstract idea conceptualized as a balance among possibilities, norms, and values, rather than a discrete entity (Harteloh, 2003; Mitchell, 2008). According to Donabedian (1990), seven attributes of healthcare define its quality: (a) efficacy: the ability of care to improve

© Springer Publishing Company DOI: 10.1891/9780826134943.0011

health, (b) effectiveness: how well health improvements are realized, (c) efficiency: the facility to obtain the best health improvement at the lowest cost, (d) optimality: balancing costs and benefits, (e) acceptability: taking into account patient preferences, (f) legitimacy: accord with social preferences concerning all of the preceding attributes, and (g) equity: fair distribution of care.

To achieve quality, it is necessary to have data-guided activities for improvement in healthcare delivery (Lynn et al., 2007) and to define and understand the issues that are hindering quality (Neuhauser, Myhre, & Alemi, 2004). These strategies include "any intervention aimed at reducing the quality gap for a group of patients representative of those encountered in routine practice" (Shojania, McDonald, Wachter, & Owens, 2004, p. 13). For example, automatic triggers can be set in an electronic medical record to remind staff to check blood glucose levels at a specific time.

Quality-improvement projects are not research studies, although they may use the scientific method. Quality-improvement projects carry no risk to patients and are meant to be generalizable only within the local setting, where the project was conducted. Research, on the other hand, is a systematic investigation meant to generate generalizable knowledge. Reinhardt and Ray (2003) proposed four criteria that distinguish a quality-improvement project from a research study:

1. Quality improvement applies research to practice; research develops new knowledge or tests new interventions.
2. There is no risk to participants in quality improvement; research could pose risk to participants.
3. The primary audience for quality improvement is the organization, and the results can be generalized only locally; research has a larger audience outside of the organization and can be generalizable to like organizations.
4. Data from quality improvement is specific to an organization; research data can be derived from multiple organizations.

Ask the following questions to determine whether the project is a research study or a quality-improvement project (Johansson, 2011; Platteborze et al., 2010):

1. Quality-improvement project—All answers should be yes for it to be a quality-improvement project:
   ■ Are patients involved only through the use of a medical record review?

- Are data being reviewed to correct deficiencies or improve a process?
- Is there a continuous monitoring process?
- Are a set of standards, benchmarks, or guidelines used for comparison?
- Is immediate feedback provided to stakeholders during and after the project?

2. Research study—All answers should be yes for it to be a research study:
   - Are interventions being tested?
   - Were patients allocated to different groups for monitoring or testing?
   - Is anyone blinded to the patients involved or the procedure or testing being done?
   - Was feedback deliberately delayed?
   - Was statistical testing done to prove or disprove a hypothesis?

DETERMINING QUALITY MEASURES

The focus of quality-improvement activities is on systems and processes that can be improved. According to Glanville, Schrim, and Wineman (2000), the classic five Ds of medical outcomes are a starting point. The five Ds are death, disease, disability, discomfort, and dissatisfaction. Examples of processes and systems amenable to quality improvement using this framework include:

- Death: Infant mortality, serious drug errors, death while under anesthesia in the operating room
- Disability: Physical, cognitive/intellectual, or developmental disabilities
- Disease: Urinary tract infections, readmission rates for heart failure (disease)
- Discomfort: Pain, pressure ulcers
- Dissatisfaction: Hospital noise levels at night, staffing mix, turnover rates, waiting times

Donabedian (2003) described three key aspects to an understanding of quality in healthcare, which can be used to determine quality indicators used for monitoring. These are structure, process, and outcomes. *Structure* is the environment in which care is provided and includes material resources (e.g., specialized equipment needed for orthopedic surgery), human resources (e.g., care provider qualifications), and organizational resources (e.g., an adequate budget). Data on structure variables are usually readily available.

Process refers to the way in which healthcare services are provided, including the individual decisions and performance of those rendering care. Process variables examine the appropriateness and completeness of care rendered. Often process variables are categorized as quality care (e.g., infection rates), safety (e.g., fall rates), or communication (e.g., discharge teaching).

Outcomes are the products that result from the interaction of structure and process. The outcome reflects what was done to a patient and how well it was done. Outcomes, as the endpoint of care, can be expected or unexpected and desirable or undesirable. Death, disability, satisfaction, length of stay, readmission rates, and cost are examples of outcome variables.

According to Donabedian (2003), examining structure, process, and outcomes as an integrated whole provides a comprehensive review of quality care. For example, when a structure, process, or outcome has been determined to be in need of improvement, it is weighted more heavily if it has one or more of the following characteristics (Health Resources and Services Administration [HRSA], 2011):

- High volume
- High frequency
- High risk
- A practice of long-standing
- Multiple unsuccessful attempts for resolution in the past
- Strong and differing opinions on cause or resolution of the problem

METHODS FOR QUALITY IMPROVEMENT

Several models exist for use in quality improvement, as presented in Table 11.1. Among these are plan-do-check-act (PDCA), Six Sigma, Baldrige, Lean, and ISO 9000. The two most frequently used are PDCA and Six Sigma.

PDCA is a four-step iterative process. The first step is to identify the problem and formulate an approach to resolving it (*plan*) by establishing objectives and expected outcomes, for example, a reduction in catheter-associated urinary tract infections or reduction in readmission rates to a detoxification facility. Second, the plan is implemented (*do*),

TABLE 11.1

QUALITY-IMPROVEMENT METHODS

Method	Key Components	Learn More
Baldridge	The Baldridge program consists of a set of 18 performance criteria divided into seven categories: 1. Leadership 2. Strategic excellence: Focus on patients 3. Other customers and markets 4. Measurement, analysis, and knowledge management 5. Workforce focus 6. Process management 7. Results	www.qualitynist.gov Flynn, B., & Saldin, B. (2001). Further evidence on the validity of the theoretical models underlying the Baldrige criteria. *Journal of Operations Management, 19*(6), 671–652.
ISO 9000	The ISO 9000 is a set of eight standards developed to result in alignment of organizational goals, communication, and continuous improvement. The standards focus on: 1. Customers 2. Leadership 3. Involvement of people 4. Process 5. Systems 6. Continual improvement 7. Factual approach to decision making 8. Supplier relationships	www.vmiso.org Sweeny, J., & Heaton, C. (2000). Interpretations and variations of ISO 9000 in acute health care. *International Journal of Quality Health Care, 12*(3), 203–209.

(continued)

TABLE 11.1 *(CONTINUED)*

QUALITY-IMPROVEMENT METHODS

Method	Key Components	Learn More
Six Sigma	Six Sigma is a quality-improvement process designed to eliminate variation, reduce the likelihood of error, and streamline processes.	www.isixsigma.org Lanham, B., & Maxson-Cooper, P. (2003). Is six sigma the answer for nursing to reduce medical errors and enhance patient safety? *Nursing Economics, 21*(1), 39–41.
Lean	The basis of Lean management is determining the value of a given process by breaking it down and identifying the value-added steps and the non–value-added steps. A central element is "stop the line," which allows any employee to stop a process when a defect is identified or suspected.	www.ihi.org/IHI/Besults/WhitePapers/GoingLeaninHealthCare.htm Furman, C., & Caplan, R. (2007). Appling the Toyota production system: Using a patient safety alert system to reduce error. *The Joint Commission Journal on Quality and Patient Safety, 33*(7), 376–386.
PDCA	PDCA is a four-step cyclical process involving establishing objectives and desired outcome, developing an implementation strategy, implementing the plan, and evaluating the results.	www.ihi.org van Tiel, F. H., Elenbaas, T. W., Voskuilen, B. M., Herczeg, J., Verheggen, F. W., Mochtar, B., & Stobberingh, E. E. (2006). Plan-do-study-act cycles as an instrument for improvement of compliance with infection control measures in care of patients after cardiothoracic surgery. *Journal of Hospital Infection, 62,* 64–70. PDCA, plan-do-check-act.

and data are collected. The do phase often incorporates such processes as Lean and Six Sigma. Lean focuses on understanding and improving processes, whereas Six Sigma seeks to uncover and reduce variation (Langley, Nolan, Nolan, Norman, & Procost, 2009). The do phase is the most extensive and time-consuming, as protocols and tools are being developed or refined, and often an educational component is necessary to instruct staff on any new processes or protocols. Third, collected data are analyzed and compared with the goals and expectations devised during the plan phase (*check*). Quality-improvement tools, such as flow charts, Pareto charts, or control charts, are used to display and interpret data. Finally, the plan is refined and further improvements are made as necessary or strategies are put into place to sustain and monitor positive outcomes (*act*). Both failures and successes are analyzed in this phase. Corrective action plans can be devised for differences in the project goals and results or a root cause analysis (RCA) can be conducted to determine major differences or lack of goal attainment.

Six Sigma is a method used to investigate operational performance improvement. It is a five-step process of defining, measuring, analyzing, improving, and controlling (DMAIC; Corn, 2009). For example, if the staff in a psychiatric rehabilitation facility believes it has a high rate of transfer to local emergency departments (EDs) for minor ailments among its residents, a team will first delineate the problem (*define*). This can be done by reviewing the transfer records of all patients taken to the ED for a specified period of time. This review will provide information on the scope of the problem, such as common reasons for transfer and cost. Second, the team will determine measures to define its success in reducing rates of transfer. Goals should be written to keep the project on track (*measure*), for example, reduce transfers to the ED by two per month over the next 6 months. Next, the team will need to analyze each of the transfers to determine the reason for each transfer and whether it were an actual emergency as well as other information that will inform development of a plan for improvement, for example, dates and times of transfer and staffing mix at times of transfer (*analyze*). Use of the quality-management tools, such as the Pareto chart, can better inform this analysis (see "Pareto Chart" section). A plan to address the process is then developed (*improve*), for example, staff education on minor versus major emergencies, review of medical coverage, or need for additional coverage (medical as well as psychiatric coverage) at certain times. Finally, the plan will need constant monitoring over time with feedback provided to staff and administrators so that progress can be monitored (*control*). Now the control chart quality-management tool can be used to monitor process control (see "Control Chart" section). This model can be used in conjunction with an RCA.

Two other frequently used strategies for quality improvement are the RCA and failure modes and effects analysis (FMEA). An RCA is a formal team investigation aimed at identifying and understanding why an event occurred. At a minimum, the team should include these members: stakeholders with decisional authority, a clinician with knowledge of the processes and procedures, and a quality-improvement expert (American Society for Quality [ASQ], 2013). An RCA is undertaken with the understanding that system issues, rather than personnel, are likely the source of an incident. According to Hughes (2008), an RCA is a labor-intensive assessment that begins after an event (e.g., a death while under anesthesia in the operating room or the suicide of a patient on a psychiatric unit) occurs. The process involves tracing and outlining the sequence of events leading to the event and putting preventive strategies into place. Meetings of the team should focus on defining and understanding the problem, brainstorming its possible causes, analyzing causes and effects, and devising a solution to the problem (ASQ, 2013). An RCA uses qualitative methods of inquiry, including interviewing those involved in the event. Interview questions are focused on enabling factors (e.g., lack of education), latent conditions (e.g., not checking the patient's identification band), and situational factors (e.g., two patients in the hospital with the same last name) that contributed to or enabled the adverse event. It is important to continually ask, "Why did this happen?" until the root cause or causes are determined. It is important to also consider events that occurred immediately prior to the event to determine whether any other factors may have contributed (The Joint Commission, 2003). The final step of an RCA is developing recommendations into a plan of corrective action.

A second commonly used strategy is an FMEA. This is an evaluation strategy used to identify and eliminate failures before they actually occur, in other words, it identifies the parts of a process that need to be strengthened or improved before an adverse event occurs. The goal of an FMEA is to prevent errors by attempting to identify the ways a process could fail, estimate the probability and consequences of each failure, and then take action to prevent the potential failures from occurring (Hughes, 2008). Brainstorming and speculation are important activities in this process. The ASQ (2013) suggests that an FMEA be considered for any of the following:

■ When a new process service is designed or implemented
■ When an existing process is used in a new way
■ When analyzing failures of an existing process
■ Periodically to monitor change over time

The focus of the analysis is on the steps in the process, failure modes (what could go wrong?), failure causes (why would the failure happen?), and failure effects (what would be the consequences of each failure?; Institute for Healthcare Improvement [IHI], 2011a). The IHI (2004) has an interactive tool to assist in conducting an FMEA. Use of this tool generates a risk score that takes into account the likelihood that the process will actually fail, the potential to detect the failure, and the severity of a failure.

TOOLS FOR QUALITY IMPROVEMENT

There are several tools that can be used to display and monitor the results of quality-improvement initiatives. The most commonly used are:

- Flow chart
- Fishbone diagram
- Control chart
- Run chart
- Pareto chart

The technique of *brainstorming*, however, is foundational to all of these improvement tools. *Brainstorming* refers to a method of discussing a problem or clinical issue in a group to generate a list of broad-ranging ideas on the topic. It is meant to be an open and creative process that uses little structure so a complete list of potential causes can be generated. All suggestions are put into a list. To be successful, a brainstorming session should have a leader who presents and clarifies the issue for discussion and one recorder (or more) who puts all ideas onto a flip chart or whiteboard. Also important to a brainstorming session is an understanding that this is not a debate on how best to address a problem, rather an open discussion of the issue. See Box 11.1 for additional details on brainstorming.

Flow Chart

A flow chart is a schematic representation of a process that allows visualization of the steps in a process. Each step is represented by a different symbol and contains a short description of the process involved in that step. Once the steps in a process are identified, the flow chart can be used to identify unnecessary or duplicative steps, missing steps, and integration among the steps. The most common types of boxes

BOX 11.1

BRAINSTORMING GUIDELINES

■ Remember that laughter and groans and even positive comments ("Great idea!") are forms of criticism.
■ Solicit as many ideas as you can.
■ Do not hold back. Crazy ideas can spark someone else's imagination and lead to creative solutions.
■ Build on someone else's idea.
■ A facilitator is needed to keep the flow of ideas going and to ensure that no ideas get lost.
■ A recorder is needed to keep track of all ideas without trying to rephrase them.
■ Keep all ideas visible. When ideas overflow to additional flip chart pages, post previous pages around the room so all ideas are still visible to everyone.

Source: Tague, R. (2004). *The quality toolbox* (2nd ed., pp. 126–127, 131–132). Milwaukee, WI: ASQ Quality Press.

seen in a flowchart are an oval, which indicates the starting and ending points of a process; a rectangle, which denotes an activity or a step in the process, and a diamond, which is a decision point. The flow chart symbols are linked together with arrows showing the direction of process flow. Flow charts can be constructed using Microsoft Excel, Word, or PowerPoint. Some common alternate names include *process flow chart, process map, process chart, process model, process flow diagram,* or just *flow diagram.* Flow charts are useful in detailing the steps of a procedure or a process, for example, how pressure ulcers are assessed (Figure 11.1).

Fishbone Diagram

A fishbone diagram is a graphic display of the possible causes or effects of a quality issue. It can be used to summarize a brainstorming session. Often, it is constructed following the development of a flow chart when all processes are understood. It can also be used following an adverse event to determine the cause of the event or to determine any potential problems in a process (RCA). Fishbones are categorized into manpower (people), material, machinery (equipment), measurement,

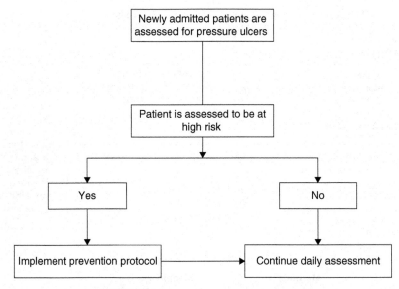

FIGURE 11.1 Flow chart example.

and methods. Environment may also be added if appropriate. Each of these categories forms a bone in the fish. Fishbone diagrams are also referred to as *cause-and-effect diagrams* or *Ishikawa diagrams* (Figure 11.2). Other areas in need of brainstorming can be added, such as environment.

Run Chart

Run charts, or line graphs, display results and variation over time and in time sequence. In a run chart, events, shown on the y-axis, are graphed against a time period on the x-axis (horizontal axis). For example, a run chart can plot the time of a written discharge order to the actual time the patient leaves the hospital room. The results might show that although the order is written in the morning, patients do not leave until late afternoon. Investigating this phenomenon could identify areas for potential improvement in the discharge process. Figure 11.3 presents a run chart used to plot the number of falls per month in order to detect whether the number is increasing, decreasing, or remaining the same over time. A general rule in interpreting a run chart is that five points in a row in either direction indicate a significant change.

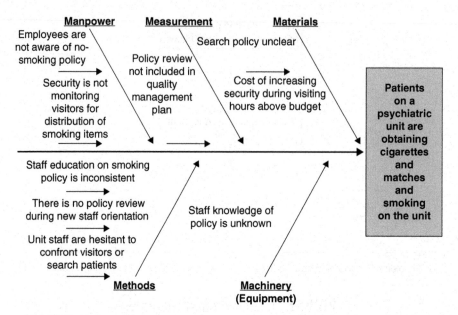

FIGURE 11.2 Fishbone diagram example indicating a violation of the no-smoking policy on a psychiatric unit.

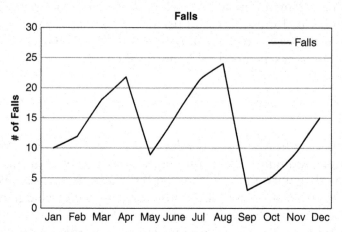

FIGURE 11.3 Run chart example.

Pareto Chart

The Pareto chart is a clustered bar chart with values arranged in order of frequency of occurrence and percentage of the total represented by each of the frequencies. A Pareto chart identifies the most significant factors in a quality issue by using the 80/20 question: *What 20% is causing 80% of a problem?* For example, although there may be many patient complaints about the food served in a hospital, a Pareto chart helps us understand what the most common complaints are and efforts to reduce complaint rates can be focused. In illustration, a hospital food service received 206 complaints about food service, which could be categorized as follows:

Complaint	Frequency
1. Food too cold	82
2. Delivered late	44
3. Tray left out of reach	26
4. Wrong order	17
5. Tasted bad	16
6. Was not delivered	10
7. Rude service	9
8. Too hot	2

Putting this information into a Pareto chart (Figure 11.4) shows that 80% of the food service complaints are related to food being delivered cold. By addressing this issue, the food service staff could meet its goal of 90% satisfaction—seen as a straight line at the top of the chart at 90 on the *x*-axis.

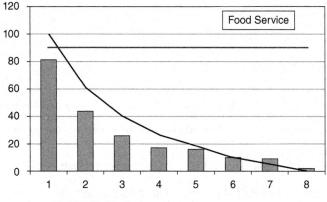

FIGURE 11.4 Pareto chart example.

Control Chart

A control chart is a graphic demonstration of statistical control of a process. *Statistical control* refers to monitoring a process over time to prevent deterioration and facilitate improvement (Wood, 2001). Basically, a control chart is a sophisticated run chart. Data are plotted over time so that patterns and trends can be easily seen. For any process, such as falls, infection rates, or readmissions, a graph displaying the central line or average of successive samples is plotted, and "control lines" are superimposed to indicate points that are "out of control."

A control chart also has three reference lines determined by historical data: a central line, which represents the average; an upper line, which represents the upper control limit; and a lower line, which represents the lower control limit. By comparing current data to the reference lines, you can assess whether the process variation is in control (consistent) or out of control (unpredictable). For example, a control chart can be used to plot the average length of time patients spend waiting before being seen at an ambulatory clinic. Figure 11.5 presents a six-quarter (18 months) view of falls. The fall rate is in control, as the mean

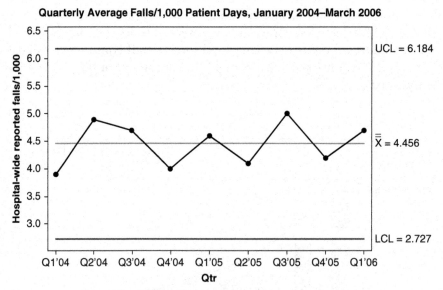

Quarterly Average Falls/1,000 Patient Days, January 2004–March 2006

LCL, lower control limit; UCL, upper control limit.

FIGURE 11.5 Control chart example.

does not extend beyond the upper and lower control limits. The value and wide-ranging use of a control chart was articulated by Stoumbous et al. (2000):

> Control charts are among the most important and widely used tools in statistics. Their applications have now moved far beyond manufacturing into engineering, environmental science, biology, genetics, epidemiology, medicine, finance, and even law enforcement and athletics. (p. 992)

Templates for a control chart and a fishbone diagram can be found at the American Society for Quality website (asq.org/learn-about-quality/quality-tools.html).

STEPS IN DEVELOPING A QUALITY-IMPROVEMENT PLAN

A quality-improvement plan serves as a guidance document that informs everyone in the organization as to the direction, timeline, activities, and importance of the quality-improvement initiative in process. An effective plan includes the following elements:

- A description of the problem to be addressed: Use as many metrics as available to establish a baseline for the problem.
- A description of quality-improvement goals and objectives: Identify the current performance for the targeted area and set goals. Goals can be related to capacity, process, or outcomes. For example, to address the problem of a high rate of readmission among heart failure patients, a new identification and referral system can be put in place. Goals would include:
  - Capacity Measure: Seventy-five percent of all direct care nursing staff will be trained on the new system for referral of heart failure patients at risk for readmission to the care transition team by the second quarter.
  - Process Measure: The care transition team will follow the PDCA cycle and focus on the extent and appropriateness of referral of at-risk heart failure patients completed in 3 months of the new referral system start date.
  - Outcome Measures: Ninety percent of patients determined to be at risk for readmission will be referred to the care transition team.

■ A description of the activities designed to meet the quality-improvement goals and objectives: Selecting the right strategy to use to address the problem is essential to success. Careful consideration of the best strategy will save time and avoid having to make adjustments once the plan is put into process. When considering strategies, identify the root cause of the problem, review any literature or documentation that details what other facilities have done when faced with similar issues, and consider available resources, including budget.

■ A description of how quality initiatives will be managed and assessed/measured: See Box 11.2.

■ A description of any necessary training: Educate the staff on the plan, both at inception and at regular intervals. Include why the

---

BOX 11.2

RESOURCES FOR MANAGING QUALITY DATA

1. Institute for Healthcare Improvement. (2011e). *Simple data collection planning.* Retrieved from http://www.ihi.org/knowledge/Pages/Tools/SimpleDataCollectionPlanning.aspx
2. Agency for Healthcare Research and Quality. (2010). *Introduction to measures of quality.* Retrieved from http://www.ahrq.gov/professionals/quality-patient-safety/quality-resources/perfmeasguide/perfmeaspt2.html
3. Agency for Healthcare Research and Quality. (2011). *National quality measures clearinghouse.* Retrieved from http://www.qualitymeasures.ahrq.gov/search/advanced-search.aspx
4. Institute for Healthcare Improvement. (2011d). *Sampling tool for quality management.* Retrieved from http://www.ihi.org/knowledge/Pages/Tools/Sampling.aspx
5. Institute for Healthcare Improvement. (2011b). *Improvement tracker.* Retrieved from http://app.ihi.org/Workspace/tracker/
6. Institute for Healthcare Improvement. (2011c). *Plan-do-study-act worksheet.* Retrieved from http://www.ihi.org/knowledge/Pages/Tools/PlanDoStudyActWorksheet.aspx
7. American Society for Quality. (2004.) *When to use a check sheet for observations.* Retrieved from http://asq.org/learn-about-quality/data-collection-analysis-tools/overview/check-sheet.html
8. Health Resources and Services Administration. (2011). *Quality management toolkit.* Retrieved from http://www.hrsa.gov/quality/toolbox/index.html

plan is being put into place, what measures are being tracked, and the staff's role in the process.

■ A description of the communication plan for quality-improvement activities and processes: Thiswill includedetails on how updates will be communicated to all staff on a regular basis.

■ A description of how improvements will be sustained in the long term is the final element of the plan.

WRITING THE QUALITY-IMPROVEMENT REPORT USING STANDARDS FOR QUALITY IMPROVEMENT REPORTING EXCELLENCE GUIDELINES

SQUIRE (Standards for Quality Improvement Reporting Excellence) guidelines were originally published in 2008 and revised in 2015 (Ogrinc et al., 2016). The guidelines address how quality-improvement efforts should be reported in professional literature; however, they are useful in writing site-specific final reports about quality improvement. See Box 11.3 for a summary of the guidelines.

BOX 11.3

SUMMARY OF SQUIRE GUIDELINES

1. Title and Abstract. Indicate in the title that this is a quality-improvement initiative. The abstract should be structured to include brief descriptions of the background, local problem, methods, interventions, results, and conclusions.
2. The introduction should describe the nature and extent of the problem, a summary of what is known about the problem, including any previous studies. A rationale for why the problem may have occurred (theories, models, concepts). This section should end with the purpose and specific aims of the initiative.
3. A description of the context in which the problem is being addressed, including members of the team is included.
4. List information on the intervention in specific detail so that it can be replicated. This information should include how data regarding the intervention was collected and measured and methods understanding variation within the data, including the effects of time as a variable.
5. A description of ethical considerations, including any conflicts of interest, need for ethics board review, and sources of funding (if applicable) is necessary.

(continued)

BOX 11.3 (CONTINUED)

6. Report the results, including associations among outcomes, interventions, and relevant contextual elements and unintended consequences such as unexpected benefits, problems, failures, or costs associated with the intervention(s). Include details about missing data.
7. Include a summary of key findings and relevance to the purpose and specific aims of the initiative.
8. Compare your results with findings from other publications and include any impact of the project on people and systems.
9. Determine the potential for generalizability of the results.
10. Include plans for sustainability.

SQUIRE, Standards for Quality Improvement Reporting Excellence.

Source: SQUIRE. (n.d.). Retrieved from http://www.squirestatement.org/index.cfm?fuseaction=Page.ViewPage&pageId=471

MEANINGFUL MEASURES

Meaningful Measures is the name of the Centers for Medicare & Medicaid Services (CMS; 2017) framework for identifying high-priority areas for quality measurement and improvement. The use of the Meaningful Measures framework encourages value through payment incentives that focus everyone's efforts on the same quality areas. The objectives of the Meaningful Measures program are to identify measures that:

1. Address high-impact measure areas that safeguard public health.
2. Are patient centered and meaningful to patients.
3. Are outcome based where possible.
4. Fulfill requirements in programs' statutes.
5. Minimize level of burden for providers.
6. Provide significant opportunity for improvement.
7. Address measures needed for population-based payment through alternative payment models.
8. Align across programs and/or with other payers (e.g., commercial payers).

Meaningful Measures are concrete quality topics that are vital to high-quality care and better patient outcomes. Examples include health-care-associated infections, prevention and treatment of opioid and other substance use disorders, and effective prevention and treatment of chronic disease. There are 16 other measures for a total of 19 Meaningful Measures as presented in Box 11.4. The CMS's strategic goal is to connect

BOX 11.4

CMS QUALITY PRIORITIES

Healthcare-associated infections

Making care safer by reducing harm caused in the delivery of care
End-of-life care according to preferences
Care is personalized and aligned with patient goals
Patient satisfaction with care
Improve or maintain patients' quality of life by addressing physical functioning
  that affects their ability to undertake daily activities most important to them
Avoid medication errors, drug interactions, and negative side effects by
  reconciling and tailoring prescriptions to meet the patient's care needs
Prevent unplanned admissions and readmissions
Promote interoperability to ensure current and useful information (i.e.,
  EMR/EHR) follows the patient and is available across every setting and
  at each healthcare interaction
Prevent diseases by providing immunizations and evidence-based screen-
  ings and by promoting healthy lifestyle behaviors and addressing maternal and child health
Promote effective management of chronic conditions, particularly for those
  with multiple chronic conditions
Diagnosis, prevention, and treatment of depression and effective management of mental disorders (e.g., schizophrenia, bipolar disorder) and
  dementia (e.g., Alzheimer's disease) with emphasis on effective integration with primary care
Ensure screening for and treatment of substance use disorders, including
  those co-occurring with mental health disorder
Reduce mortality rate for patients in all healthcare settings
Ensure high-quality and timely care with equal access for all patients and
  consumers
Increase the use and quality of home- and community-based services to
  promote public health, including a focus on health literacy
Ensure patients receive the care they need while avoiding unnecessary tests
  and procedures
Improve care by optimizing health outcomes and resource use associated
  with treating acute clinical conditions or procedures
Ensure high-quality and timely care with equal access for all patients and
  consumers, including those with social risk factors, for all health episodes in all settings of care
CMS, Centers for Medicare & Medicaid Services; EHR, electronic health
  record; EMR, electronic medical record.

Source: cms.gov

these measures to six cross-cutting criteria: eliminate disparities, track measurable outcomes, safeguard public health, achieve cost savings, improve access to rural communities, and reduce burden. Each of these overall priority measures has a subset of measures. For example, one of the Meaningful Meausures priorities is "Promote Effective Prevention and Treatment of Chronic Disease", which has five submeasures: Preventive Care; Management of Chronic Conditions; Prevention, Treatment, and Management of Mental Health; Prevention and Treatment of Opioid and Substance Use Disorders; and Risk-Adjusted Mortality.

CONCLUSIONS

To carry out a quality-improvement project requires thought and attention to detail. Significant time needs to be devoted to the specific aims and expected measurable outcomes of the project. Without such attention to detail, the project will lack focus. Clancy (2010) discussed seven mainstays of a safer healthcare system. Attention to any of these can form the basis of a quality-improvement project:

- Report near misses and other adverse events.
- Take corrective action steps to prevent future incidents from happening again.
- Communicate errors to patients.
- Apologize and waive hospital and physicians' fees when an error or other mishap occurs.
- Bridge systemic gaps that contribute to adverse events.
- Collect data and measure performance to determine whether improvements have been made.
- Educate and train staff on patient safety.

■ QUESTIONS FOR DISCUSSION

1. Describe any quality-improvement activities you have conducted.
2. Review the CMS' list of Meaningful Measures. Discuss how these are being addressed in your work setting.
3. Review the issue depicted in Figure 11.2, which exemplifies the fishbone diagram. What strategies would you put into place to address this issue? How would you monitor and sustain your strategies?
4. The "study" phase of the PDSA cycle is focued on understanding the data you collect and deciding how to display that data for

maximum impact. In the link that follows you will see a 25-minute presentation on how to display data over time using a run chart and how to display the data in subgroups. How comfortable are you with this approach? What do you need to know?

app.ihi.org/lms/lessondetailview.aspx?LessonGUID=7ea95efc -454f-44a9-a0d0-b70a0152e1e8&CourseGUID=7ab177dc -a9cf-4d1d-b870-f4be6e8d8f67&CatalogGUID=4cc435f0 -d43b-4381-84b8-899b35082938

■ REFLECTIVE EXERCISES

1. Think about a clinical problem you want to improve, for example, reduce length of stay, lower readmission and fall rates, adjust

---

EXAMPLES OF QUALITY-IMPROVEMENT PROJECTS

Evaluating Fundamentals of Care: The Development of a Unit-Level Quality Measurement and Improvement Program

The project aimed to develop a unit-level quality measurement and improvement program using evidence-based fundamentals of care. Feedback from patients, families, and staff, coupled with audit data from 2014, indicated variability in the delivery of fundamental aspects of care, such as monitoring, nutrition, pain management, and environmental cleanliness. A general inductive approach was used to explore the fundamentals of care and design a measurement and improvement program. Five phases were used to explore the evidence and design and test a measurement and improvement framework. Nine identified fundamental elements of care were used to define expected standards of care and develop and test a measurement and improvement framework. Four peer reviews conducted every 6 months have been undertaken since June 2015. Charge nurse managers used results to identify quality improvements. Significant improvement was demonstrated overall in six of the 27 units, for seven of the nine standards and three of the four measures. In all, 89% ($n = 24$) of units improved their overall result.

Reference

Parr, J. M., Bell, J., & Koziol-McLain, J. (2018). Evaluating fundamentals of care: The development of a unit-level quality measurement and improvement programme. *Journal of Clinical Nursing*. Epub ahead of print January 2. doi:10.1111/jocn.14250

Utilization of a Nurse-Driven Protocol to Decrease Catheter-Associated Urinary Tract Infections

The purpose of this project was to develop a nurse-driven protocol that allows nurses to remove urinary catheters without a physician's order and monitor

(continued)

EXAMPLES OF QUALITY-IMPROVEMENT PROJECTS (*CONTINUED*)

the use of the protocol over a 5-month period. This was a quality-improvement study using a PDCA cycle. The protocol was designed by a multidisciplinary group after the review of the literature (plan). Numerous revisions were carried out to the protocol based on input from managers, advanced practice nurses, staff nurses, physicians, and various hospital practice committees. After the protocol was approved, tools for training for educational sessions were developed by four advanced practice nurses. Education consisted of a variety of formats, including online learning, information sheets posted in the units, and face-to-face learning (do). Compliance in using the protocol was monitored during multidisciplinary rounds, which were conducted daily. Data were collected on the prevalence of urinary catheters as well as the rate of catheter-associated urinary tract infections prior to the implementation of the nurse-driven protocol. Data were also collected on the prevalence of urinary catheters as well as the rate of catheter-associated urinary tract infections for 5 months after the implementation of the nurse-driven protocol. The data-analysis method consisted of an independent samples two-tailed t-test. This study compared one sample (preprotocol) to another sample (postprotocol) to see whether there was a decrease in the number of urinary catheters used in the ICU and the rate of hospital-wide catheter-associated urinary tract infections postintervention (check). Data analysis revealed that the mean infection rate for the preprotocol group (N = 6463) was 1.231; the mean rate for the postprotocol group (N = 5167) was 0.348. This decrease in infection rate in the postintervention group is calculated to have a 95% confidence interval and is statistically significant with a p value of less than .0001. In looking at the ICU's catheter utilization ratio, the utilization ratio of catheters decreased. The power of this study was calculated to be less than .0001. Given the high power of the study, as well as a 95% confidence interval, the project does demonstrate that a nurse-driven protocol allowing nurses to remove urinary catheters without a physician order does decrease the number of urinary catheter days as well as the rate of urinary tract infections in a community hospital. These measures will continue to be monitored and reported back to staff to sustain these lower rates (act). By allowing nurses to carry out the process of removing urinary catheters without a physician's order, the hospital gains through future increases in value-based purchasing incentives as well as by not being penalized financially for urinary tract infections. However, the biggest advantage lies with the improvement in patient care in terms of a decreased morbidity, mortality, pain, and suffering related to a catheter-associated urinary tract infection.

Reference

Barto, D. (2011). *Utilization of a nurse driven protocol to decrease catheter associated urinary tract infections.* In C. Holly (Ed.), *Scholarly inquiry and the DNP capstone* (p. 153). New York, NY: Springer Publishing.

operating room start times, address the issue of nurse retention, adjust staffing mix, or reduce infection rates.
- Who will be on your team?
- What data will you need to implement your project?
- Where can that data be found?
- How will you collect the data that you need?
- What is the timeline for the project?
- How will you display the data?
- How will you disseminate the data?

2. Attend a quality-improvement committee meeting. Answer the following questions:
- Who are the members of the committee?
- What quality-improvement method are they using?
- What quality indicators are they discussing?
- What information are they using to inform their discussions?
- What are the outcomes of the discussion?

■ SUGGESTED READINGS

Hain, D. (2017). Exploring the evidence. Focusing on the fundamentals: Comparing and contrasting nursing research and quality improvement. *Nephrology Nursing Journal, 44*(6), 541–544.

Porter, R., Cullen, L., Farrington, M., Matthews, G., & Tucker, S. (2018). Original research exploring clinicians' perceptions about sustaining an evidence-based fall prevention program. *American Journal of Nursing, 118*(5), 24–33. doi:10.1097/01.NAJ .0000532806.35972.29

Rholdon, R. (2017). Outcomes of a quality improvement project: An implementation of inpatient infant safe sleep practices. *Pediatric Nursing, 43*(5), 229–232.

Rooney, J. J., & Vanden Heuvel, L. N. (2004). Root cause analysis for beginners. *Quality Process.* Retrieved from http://asq.org/qic/display-item/index.html?item=19550

Stausmire, J., & Ulrich, C. (2015). Making it meaningful: Finding quality improvement projects worthy of your time, effort, and expertise. *Critical Care Nurse, 35*(6), 57–62. doi:10.4037/ccn2015232

Wells, S., Tamir, O., Gray, J., Naidoo, D., Bekhit, M., & Goldmann, D. (2018). Are quality improvement collaboratives effective? A systematic review. *BMJ Quality & Safety, 3,* 226–240. doi:10.1136/bmjqs-2017-006926

REFERENCES

Agency for Healthcare Research and Quality. (2010). *Introduction to measures of quality.* Retrieved from http://www.ahrq.gov/professionals/quality-patient-safety/quality-resources /perfmeasguide/perfmeaspt2.html

Agency for Healthcare Research and Quality. (2011). *National quality measures clearinghouse.* Retrieved from http://www.qualitymeasures.ahrq.gov/search/advanced-search.aspx

American Society for Quality. (2004). *When to use a check sheet for observations*. Retrieved from http://asq.org/learn-about-quality/data-collection-analysis-tools/overview/check-sheet .html

American Society for Quality. (2013). Retrieved from https://videos.asq.org/root-cause -analysis

Barto, D. (2011). Utilization of a nurse driven protocol to decrease catheter associated urinary tract infections. In C. Holly (Ed.), *Scholarly inquiry and the DNP capstone* (p. 153). New York, NY: Springer Publishing.

Centers for Medicare & Medicaid Services. (2017). Meaningful measures hub. Retrieved from https://www.cms.gov/Medicare/Quality-Initiatives-Patient-Assessment-Instruments /QualityInitiativesGenInfo/MMF/General-info-Sub-Page.html

Clancy, C. M. (2010). *Patient safety and medical liability reform: Putting the patient first.* Retrieved from www.psqh.com/analysis/september-october-201016/

Corn, J. B. (2009). Six sigma in health care. *Radiologic Technology, 81*(1), 92–95.

Donabedian, A. (1990). The seven pillars of quality. *Archives of Pathology & Laboratory Medicine, 114*(11), 1115–1118.

Donabedian, A. (2003). *An introduction to quality assurance in healthcare*. New York, NY: Oxford University Press.

Flynn, B., & Saldin, B. (2001). Further evidence on the validity of the theoretical models underlying the Baldrige criteria. *Journal of Operations Management, 19*(6), 671–652.

Furman, C., & Caplan, R. (2007). Appling the Toyota production system: Using a patient safety alert system to reduce error. *The Joint Commission Journal on Quality and Patient Safety, 33*(7), 376–386.

Glanville, I., Schirm, V., & Wineman, N. M. (2000). Using evidence-based practice for managing clinical outcomes in advanced practice nursing. *Journal of Nursing Care Quality, 15*(1), 1–11. doi:10.1097/00001786-200010000-00002

Harteloh, P. P. M. (2003). The meaning of quality in health care: A conceptual analysis. *Health Care Analysis, 11*(3), 259–267. doi:10.1023/B:HCAN.0000005497.53458.ef

Health Resources and Services Administration. (2011). *Quality management toolkit.* Retrieved from http://www.hrsa.gov/quality/toolbox/index.html

Hughes, R. G. (2008). Tools and strategies for quality improvement and patient safety. In, R. G. Hughes (Ed.), *Patient safety and quality: An evidence-based handbook for nurses*. Rockville, MD: Agency for Healthcare Research and Quality. Retrieved from www.ncbi .nlm.nih.gov/books/NBK2682/

Institute for Healthcare Improvement. (2004). *Failure modes and effects analysis*. Retrieved from http://www.ihi.org/knowledge/Pages/Tools/FailureModesandEffectsAnalysisTool .aspx

Institute for Healthcare Improvement. (2011a). *Failure modes and effects analysis tool*. Retrieved from http://www.ihi.org/knowledge/Pages/Tools/FailureModesandEffects AnalysisTool.aspx

Institute for Healthcare Improvement. (2011b). *Improvement tracker*. Retrieved from http://app.ihi.org/Workspace/tracker

Institute for Healthcare Improvement. (2011c). *Plan-do-study-act worksheet*. Retrieved from http://www.ihi.org/knowledge/Pages/Tools/PlanDoStudyActWorksheet.aspx

Institute for Healthcare Improvement. (2011d). *Sampling tool for quality management*. Retrieved from http://www.ihi.org/knowledge/Pages/Tools/Sampling.aspx

Institute for Healthcare Improvement. (2011e). *Simple data collection planning*. Retrieved from http://www.ihi.org/knowledge/Pages/Tools/SimpleDataCollectionPlanning.aspx

Johansson, A. C. (2011). Perspective: medical education research and the institutional review board; reexamining the process. *Academic Medicine, 86*, 809–817. doi:10.1097/ ACM.0b013e31821d6c4c

Langley, G., Nolan, K., Nolan, T., Norman, C., & Procost, L. (2009). *The improvement guide: A practical approach to enhancing organizational performance* (2nd ed.). San Francisco, CA: Jossey-Bass.

Lanham, B., & Maxson-Cooper, P. (2003). Is six sigma the answer for nursing to reduce medical errors and enhance patient safety? *Nursing Economics, 21*(1), 39–41.

Lynn, J., Baily, M. A., Bottrell, M., Jennings, B., Levine, R. J., Davidoff, F., . . . James, B. (2007). The ethics of using quality improvement methods in health care. *Annals of Internal Medicine, 146*, 666–673. doi:10.7326/0003-4819-146-9-200705010-00155

Mitchell, P. (2008). Defining patient safety and quality care. In, R. G. Hughes (Ed.), *Patient safety and quality: An evidence-based handbook for nurses*. Rockville, MD: Agency for Healthcare Research and Quality. Retrieved from www.ncbi.nlm.nih.gov/books/NBK2681/

Neuhauser, D., Myhre, S., & Alemi, F. (2004). *Personal continuous quality improvement workbook* (7th ed.). Washington, DC: Academy for Healthcare Improvement. Retrieved from http://www.a4hi.org/docs/Neuhauser_personal_improvement_project_workbook.pdf

Ogrinc, G., Davies, L., Goodman D, Batalden, P., Davidoff, F., & Stevens, D. (2016) SQUIRE 2.0 (Standards for Quality Improvement Reporting Excellence): Revised publication guidelines from a detailed consensus process. *BMJ Quality & Safety, 25*(12), 986–992. doi:10.1136/bmjqs-2015-004411

Parr, J. M., Bell, J., & Koziol-McLain, J. (2018). Evaluating fundamentals of care: The development of a unit-level quality measurement and improvement programme. *Journal of Clinical Nursing*. Epub ahead of print January 2. doi:10.1111/jocn.14250

Platteborze, L., Young-McCaughan, S., King-Letzkus, I., McClinton, A., Halliday, A., & Jefferson, T. C. (2010). Performance improvement/research advisory panel: A model for determining whether a project is a performance or quality improvement activity or research. *Military Medicine, 175*, 290–291. doi:10.7205/MILMED-D-09-00087

Reinhardt, A. C., & Ray, L. N. (2003). Differentiating quality improvement from research. *Applied Nursing Research, 16*(1), 2–8. doi:10.1053/apnr.2003.50000

Shojania, K. G., McDonald, K. M., Wachter, R. M., & Owens, D. K. (2004). *Closing the quality gap: A critical analysis of quality improvement strategies, Volume 1–Series Overview and Methodology Technical Review 9* (Contract No 290-02-0017 to the Stanford University–UCSF Evidence-based Practice Center). Rockville, MD: Agency for Healthcare Research and Quality. AHRQ Publication No. 04-0051–1.

Standards for Quality Improvement Reporting Excellence. (n.d.). Retrieved from http://www.squirestatement.org/index.cfm?fuseaction=Page.ViewPage&pageId=471

Stoumbous, Z. G., Reynolds, M. R. Jr, Ryan, T. P., & Woodall, W. H. (2000). The state of statistical process control as we proceed into the 21st century. *Journal of the American Statistical Association, 95*(451), 992–998. doi:10.1080/01621459.2000.10474292

Sweeny, J., & Heaton, C. (2000). Interpretations and variations of ISO 9000 in acute health care. *International Journal of Quality Health Care, 12*(3), 203–209.

Tague, R. (2004). *The quality toolbox* (2nd ed., pp. 126–127, 131–132). Milwaukee, WI: ASQ Quality Press.

The Joint Commission. (2003). Using aggregate root cause analysis to improve patient safety. The *Joint Commission Journal on Quality and Patient, 29*(8), 434–439.

van Tiel, F. H., Elenbaas, T. W., Voskuilen, B. M., Herczeg, J., Verheggen, F. W., Mochtar, B., & Stobberingh, E. E. (2006). Plan-do-study-act cycles as an instrument for improvement of compliance with infection control measures in care of patients after cardiothoracic surgery. *Journal of Hospital Infection, 62*, 64–70.

Wood, M. (2001). Statistical process monitoring in the 21st century. In J. Antony & D. Preece (Eds.), *Understanding, managing & implementing quality* (pp. 103–121). London, UK: Routledge.

CHAPTER 12

Program Evaluation

OBJECTIVES

At the end of the chapter, you will be able to:

- Define *program evaluation*.
- Differentiate among goal-based, process, outcome, formative, and summative evaluations.
- Write evaluation goals.
- Develop an evaluation plan.

KEY CONCEPTS

Most evaluations fall into one of five categories:

- Formative evaluation is structured to provide information for immediate project improvement.
- Summative evaluation is conducted to determine accountability, which requires determining the overall effectiveness or merit and worth of an object under evaluation.
- Outcome evaluation is used to measure whether the project achieved its intended outcome.
- Goal-based evaluation is used to determine the extent to which programs are meeting predetermined goals or objectives.
- Process-based evaluation focuses on developing a complete understanding of how a program works.

Every evaluation is different, as it is guided by the specific purpose of the evaluation, the evaluation questions asked, and the developmental stage of the program. An important point to remember is that program evaluation is conducted to improve practice.

© Springer Publishing Company DOI: 10.1891/9780826134943.0012   211

INTRODUCTION

Evaluation involves a critical examination that ultimately demonstrates a program's progress. Program evaluation provides a structured method of collecting and analyzing information about a program's activities, characteristics, and outcomes using valid and reliable methods to examine the process or outcomes of an organization (Grinnel & Unrae 2008). According to Patton (2008), *program evaluation* is the "systematic collection of information about the activities, characteristics, and results of programs to make judgments about the program" (p. 39), whereas Rossi, Lipsey, and Freeman (2004) believe that evaluation is a method of social research designed to answer questions of policy. Typically, evaluation involves assessment of one of the following: (a) program need, (b) program plan, (c) program performance, (d) program impact, or (e) program effectiveness. The motivation for conducting a program evaluation is to show the success and benefits of an approach and to determine a program's quality. The purpose of an evaluation can be accountability or program development (Centers for Disease Control and Prevention [CDC], 2011; Patton, 2008).

A carefully planned and conducted program evaluation can:

1. Answer such questions as, "Is the program having its intended effect?" "How can it be improved?" and "Are there better and more cost-effective options to run the program?"
2. Identify program strengths and weaknesses to improve or strengthen the program.
3. Produce data or verify results that can be used to expand the program.
4. Produce valid comparisons between programs to decide which should be retained in the face of pending budget cuts.
5. Describe effective programs for duplication elsewhere.

GUIDING PRINCIPLES OF EVALUATION

The American Evaluation Association (2013) has developed a set of guidelines for the design and conduct of evaluation activities (www.eval.org/GPTraining/GP%20Training%20Final/gp.principles.pdf). These include that the evaluation should:

■ Address both the strengths and weaknesses of the program.
■ Demonstrate cultural competence in the selection of evaluation strategies.

- Report any real or potential conflicts of interest regarding the evaluation.
- Seek a comprehensive understanding of the contextual elements of the evaluation.
- Abide by current professional ethics standards and regulations regarding confidentiality, informed consent, and protection of human subjects.
- Seek to maximize the benefits and reduce any harm that might occur from an evaluation.

An important principle maintains that evaluators should possess the appropriate knowledge and skill to conduct an evaluation. These include having an understanding of research methods and analysis, the ability to think critically and make judgments based on findings, and the capacity to move beyond superficial information to understand fully how a program operates.

Evaluation should be practical and feasible and conducted within consideration of certain parameters:resources, time, and political context. Evaluation findings should be used to make decisions about program implementation and to improve program effectiveness. In this way, program evaluation is different from research, in that a research

TABLE 12.1

RESEARCH VERSUS PROGRAM EVALUATION

	Research	Program Evaluation
Purpose	Test hypothesis or generate meaning	Achieve greater or enhanced understanding
Guiding questions	Facts: Provide descriptions, associations, effects Meaning	Value: Determine program merit, worth, significance, quality, cost
Strengths	Internal validity (accuracy, precision) External validity (generalizability)	Context Utility
Use	Is disseminated to interested audiences	Provides feedback to stakeholders

Source: Adapted from MacDonald, G., Starr, G., Schooley, M., Yee, S. L., Klimowski, K., & Turner, K. (2001). Introduction to program evaluation for comprehensive tobacco control programs. Atlanta, GA: Centers for Disease Control and Prevention. Retrieved from http://www.cdc.gov/tobacco/tobacco_control_programs/surveillance_evaluation/evaluation_manual/pdfs/evaluation.pdf

study is conducted to test a hypothesis or generate meaning, whereas a program evaluation is conducted to improve practice (MacDonald et al, 2001). Table 12.1 displays some of the principles that distinguish program evaluation from research.

TYPES OF EVALUATION

Evaluations fall into one of two broad categories: formative and summative. Formative evaluations are conducted during program development and implementation. Formative evaluation results are used to understand and plan for the best ways to achieve program goals. Summative evaluations are completed when a program is established. Summative evaluation results can reveal the extent to which a program is meetings its goals.

Formative Evaluation

Formative evaluation is structured to provide information for project improvement. Emphasis is on findings that are timely, concrete, and immediately useful (Rossi et al., 2004). The purpose of a formative evaluation is to better *form* the program to meet its expected outcomes. A formative evaluation allows consideration and review of program planning efforts while in the early stages of implementation, rather than waiting until the program has been fully developed and completed. Also known as a *usability study*, a formative evaluation can uncover unintended consequences. For example, Landau (2001) provides two examples of unintended results of a program identified during a formative evaluation: one negative and one positive. First, she explains that during the early days of antidrug films, young people learned new ways of drug use by watching movies that illustrated behavior that was intended to discourage drug use. On a more positive note, she described that while television stations, under the Americans With Disabilities Act, provide closed-captioned programming to make broadcasts accessible to people who are hearing impaired or deaf, these captions are also used by those who are just learning to read or who are learning a second language.

Formative evaluation as applied to healthcare programs may be not appropriate for evaluating all healthcare programs. Stetler et al. (2006), for example, explain that in a randomized controlled trial, researchers do not typically change or modify the experimental arm once it has been approved; however, changes in a quality-improvement project as it is being conducted may be important in obtaining the right data essential to improving processes, which is the purpose of a formative evaluation.

Formative evaluation differs from the other types of evaluation, as it is ongoing and involves an informed judgment on the part of the evaluator as to whether the program is likely to meet its intended goals (Beyer, 1995). Formative evaluation can include a needs assessment, which allows a determination of who needs the program, how great the need is, and what can be done to best meet the need. A needs assessment can also provide insight into what characteristics new programs should have to meet stakeholder needs. For example, Pennel, McLeroy, Burdine, and Matarrita-Cascanate (2015) conducted a community health needs assessment (CHNA) to better understand how nonprofit hospitals are fulfilling the CHNA provision of the 2010 Patient Protection and Affordable Care Act, information that could be used to improve community health programs.

Considerations in planning a formative evaluation include:

■ Plan the evaluation before development of the program is completed.
■ Conduct the formative evaluation several times during the program development phase.
■ Focus on the collection of information that will be of immediate use when planning and developing the program.
■ Use the results of each evaluation to revise or modify the program (Beyer, 1995).

Summative Evaluation

Summative evaluation provides a summary. It is retrospective in nature in contrast to the prospective view needed for a formative evaluation. Summative evaluation determines whether an intervention, service, or program is working. Summative evaluation takes place most often at the end of a project. As such, summative evaluation is referred to as *ex-post evaluation* (after the event) and is linked to accountability. Summative evaluation can be one of two types— outcome or impact—or a combination of the two forms.

Outcome evaluation examines the extent to which a program is meeting its goals and objectives. Outcomes can be short term or long term. For example, an improvement in patient knowledge of diabetes self-care management strategies may be a short-term goal prior to discharge with a change in hemoglobin A1C (HgA1C) levels a longer goal.

Impact evaluation determines whether broad, long-term change has occurred because of the program. An impact evaluation may focus on a community or school as well as the human impact the program offers. For example, a summative evaluation on impact is about the decreased rates and sustainability of smoking following a smoking-cessation program, rather than a description of how many attended the program and demonstrated increased knowledge about the hazards of smoking.

Some reasons to undertake a summative evaluation include (Evaluation Toolbox, 2010):

- To determine whether a project or program has met its goals/ objectives/outcomes
- To determine the impact of a program
- To compare the impact of different projects and make decisions on future spending allocation
- To develop a better understanding of the process of change, to find out what works, what doesn't, and why; this provides the knowledge to improve future projects and implementation efforts
- To determine whether a program is still operating as originally intended

Goal-Based Evaluation

Goal-based evaluations determine the extent to which programs are meeting predetermined goals or objectives. Goal-based evaluation does not question whether the selected goals are legitimate; it determines whether the goal, as stated, has been met (Evaluation Toolbox, 2010). A goal-based evaluation can be either formative or summative.

A goal is a statement that can be used to ascertain an organization's progress. Goals can be related to money, equipment, facilities, staffing, timelines, or other resources. Setting goals provides a purpose and a focus for action. A goal is a global statement of what is to be accomplished and it may have subordinate, more focused goals attached to it. Goals should be written in a positive manner using the future tense, provide a time frame for accomplishment, and be clear in what is intended. The three Ps of a good goal are that they are positive, precise, and performance oriented.

Examples of program goals are:

- At the end of one year, $500,000 for program operations will have been awarded.
- Six months following completion of a smoking-cessation program, 50% of participants will have stopped smoking.
- Emergency department wait times will have decreased to 15 minutes or less by the end of the year.

Goal-based evaluation does not question whether the goals are valid, nor whether appropriate measures of effectiveness are being assessed. A goal-based evaluation just determines whether the goals are being met.

Process Evaluation

Process or implementation evaluation is focused on a complete understanding of how a program works. It is useful when replicating the program in other settings and for monitoring a program's effectiveness. Process evaluation is the most commonly used method of evaluation, as it can be used as a stand-alone form of assessment or in combination with an outcome evaluation. A process evaluation answers the question, "Does the program deliver its intended objectives to the target population?" (Rossi et al., 2004). Basically, a process evaluation assesses the fidelity (faithfulness to the original intent) and effectiveness (degree of success in producing a desired result) of a program's implementation. According to Rossi et al. (2004),

> (a process evaluation) might examine how consistently services actually delivered are consistent with the goals of the program, whether services are delivered to appropriate recipients, how will service delivery be organized, the effectiveness of program management, the use of program resources, and other such matters. (p. 57)

Process evaluation focuses on the internal operations of a program to determine its strengths and weaknesses and areas needing improvement. A process evaluation can map an actual operation, for example, the discharge process or the experiences of families in the ICU. It is a search for patterns, trends, successes, and failures (Patton, 2008). For example, Plochg, Delnoij, van der Kruk, Janmaat, and Klazinga (2005) evaluated the process of an intermediate care model between a university hospital and a residential home using t-tests and chi-squared test to assess significance. Semistructured interviews were conducted with 21 staff members representing all disciplines. Results indicated that despite high expectations, a heterogeneous, more-complex-than-expected patient population, an unqualified staff, and cultural differences between collaborating partners impeded implementation. The evaluators concluded that setting up a discharge model of intermediate care between a university hospital and a residential home is less straightforward than was originally perceived.

Outcomes-Based Evaluation

Outcome or impact evaluation can be conducted for one outcome or as part of a summative evaluation of all outcomes. For example, the impact of a state-wide media campaign for youth suicide prevention was analyzed through call volumes to a national hotline, to determine whether the advertisements have raised awareness of the hotline (one goal: increased calls to the hotline (Jenner, Jenner, Matthews-Sterling, Butts, & Evans Williams, 2010).

In an outcome evaluation, efforts focus on a single program. Such analysis cannot be attempted without the baseline data for comparison. For example, in a heart failure program, two outcomes measures were chosen, and they were monitored before and after the implementation of the program. The measures were:

1. The patient discharged with a diagnosis of heart failure will see a primary care provider within 2 weeks of discharge.
2. Patients discharged with a diagnosis of heart failure will not be readmitted for the same diagnosis within a 90-day period.

Program success was defined as whether, or to what extent, these two goals were met. Other approaches to basic outcome evaluation might include comparisons within a program. For example, what are the characteristics of those who were not followed up by a primary care provider within a 2-week period or who were readmitted with the same diagnosis within 90 days of discharge? This extension of the outcome evaluation can predict those at high risk at the outset of the program and follow-up efforts can be focused.

The value of an outcome evaluation lies in its ability to provide information regarding program performance using before-and-after comparisons. It allows the evaluator to answer the question, "Did the program make a difference?" Although it doesn't explain what would happen if the program was not implemented, it provides information regarding the program's impact on preselected criteria. Hendricks, Plantz, and Pritchard (2008) provides an excellent overview of outcomes-based evaluation, including introduction to outcomes measurement, a program outcome model, reasons to measure outcomes, and use of program outcome findings.

DEVELOPING AN EVALUATION PLAN

An evaluation plan is a document that outlines the way in which the evaluation will be conducted. The CDC (2011) has developed a framework for writing an evaluation plan that involves engaging stakeholders, describing the program, focusing on the evaluation design, gathering credible evidence, justifying conclusions, and disseminating them to ensure use of the findings.

The first step in any program evaluation is to determine the goals of the evaluation and write the questions that the evaluation is designed to answer. In other words, what are you going to evaluate? These questions will determine the type of evaluation to be conducted. For example, if the intent of the evaluation is to determine how a program works, then a process evaluation is appropriate. A selective focus for the evaluation is usually necessary because an evaluation of an entire program (a formative evaluation) is costly and time intensive. For example, the evaluation may address teaching style, patient satisfaction, or more complex behavioral changes related to a specific intervention. Whatever the focus of the evaluation, it is necessary to write goals and questions that guide the process.

The SMART model provides a framework for developing evaluation goals. Goals should be *s*pecific, *m*easurable, *a*chievable, *r*esults focused, and *t*imely. In other words, *SMART*. To be specific, goals should be precise and simple and clearly define what will be accomplished. They should be jargon free and have only one meaning. To be measurable, audit criteria should be quantifiable so that tangible evidence of accomplishments is obtained. Achievable goals are those that are possible and practical. Goals should measure results or outcomes, rather than activities. Timely audit criteria are those that have a specified time frame for accomplishment, such as daily, upon admission, quarterly, or annually. Goals should be linked to a time frame (Holly, Rittenmeyer, & Weeks, 2014). Evaluation questions should be specific to the intent of the evaluation. See Table 12.2 for examples on how to focus an evaluation question. Other considerations when writing the evaluation plan are:

■ What information is needed to answer the evaluation questions?
■ Where will the information be found?
■ What are the methods for collecting information? To answer the evaluation questions, the right data need to be collected. Table 12.3 provides an overview of the commonly used evaluative data-collection methods. It is useful to develop a plan for the collection of data that details the information needed and its source for each of the evaluation questions (Table 12.4). Both quantitative and qualitative data are collected for a program evaluation. The use of both types of data, in combination, provides both a measure of change and important contextual information. Some considerations when collecting data for evaluation include the

TABLE 12.2

FOCUSING EVALUATION QUESTIONS	
Type of Evaluation	Focus
Outcome/impact evaluation	What do people do differently as a result of the program? What are the strengths and weaknesses of the program? Did the program reach its intended audience?
Process evaluation	What methods were used to deliver the program? Were resources adequate to meet program goals?
Goal-based evaluation	Were intended goals met? Do goals have to be refined?
Formative evaluation	Who benefited from the program? What lessons can be learned from this initiative? Is the program sustainable?

TABLE 12.3

CHARACTERISTICS OF COMMONLY USED METHODS OF DATA COLLECTION FOR PROGRAM EVALUATION	
Method	Characteristics
Questionnaire	Nonthreatening Anonymous Inexpensive Information can be obtained from a large sample
Interviews/focus groups	Time-consuming Provides in-depth information about processes, procedures, and conditions
Document review	Uses patient care records, meeting minutes, financial records, and status reports to determine how a program operates
Observation	Time-consuming Examinesf a program in operation

TABLE 12.4

DATA-COLLECTION PLAN

Evaluation Question	Outcome/Goal or Indicator	Information Needed	Data Source	Method of Data Collection	Frequency of Data Collection	Responsible Party
What do you want to know?	How will you know it?	What do you need to know?	Where can you find this data?	How will you collect the data you need?	How often will you collect the needed data?	Who will be in charge of making sure the data is collected and analyzed?
How well is the suicide hotline program working?	Call volume will increase by 20% in 3 months	Number of calls before and after implementation of a media campaign for prevention of suicide	Electronic call registry	Retrospective review of call registry	Aggregated weekly	Program director

Source: Adapted from Centers for Disease Control and Prevention. (2011). *Developing an effective evaluation plan.* Atlanta, GA: Centers for Disease Control and Prevention, National Center for Chronic Disease Prevention and Health Promotion, Office on Smoking and Health; Division of Nutrition, Physical Activity, and Obesity. Retrieved from http://www.cdc.gov/obesity/downloads/CDC-Evaluation-Workbook-508.pdf; Jenner, E., Jenner, L.W., Matthews-Sterling, M.. Butts, J., & Evans Williams, T. (2010). Awareness effects of a youth suicide prevention media campaign in Louisiana. *Suicide and Life-Threatening Behavior, 40*(4), 394–406. doi:10.1521/suli.2010.40.4.394

following: (a) Both qualitative and quantitative data are collected so that all aspects of the program can be understood, and (b) the entire program needs to be evaluated. A snapshot is not adequate (Evaluation Toolbox, 2010).

■ What is the time frame for collecting information? That is, when will the evaluation period start and when will it end? This time frame is the period during which you will collect data to answer the question, for example, 3 months, 6 months, or 1 year.

■ How will the information will be analyzed? Analysis of the quantitative and qualitative data collected should follow the accepted methods for the type of data collected; for example, interview or focus data should be analyzed using content analysis. When analyzing data for a program evaluation, the analysis is focused on the purpose and goals of the evaluation. For example, if the intent of the evaluation is to identify strengths and weaknesses, data should be organized by results related to strengths and weaknesses of the program (Grinnel & Unrae, 2008).

■ Who will get the evaluation report?

THE EVALUATION REPORT

Evaluation reports begin with an executive summary. An executive summary is a one-page description of the main findings of the evaluation. It is an extended abstract that describes the important points and findings of the evaluation and includes a clear description of the program, service, or intervention being evaluated; a statement of the purpose of the evaluation; a brief description of methods used for data collection and analysis. The major findings and conclusions linked to the evaluation goals should also be included in the executive summary. Although there is no length requirement for an executive summary, a good summary will be at least two single-spaced pages.

The remainder of the report provides extended detail for each of the sections of the executive summary, including:

1. The purpose of the report and the type of evaluation conducted should be explained in some detail so that the reader understands the process used.
2. Detailed information is given on the background and history of the program, service, or intervention that was evaluated.
3. The report describes the goals of the evaluation or the questions it answers.

4. A methods section describes the information collected, including any tools used to collect the information and how the data were analyzed

5. Interpretations and conclusions: These should be as transparent as possible. An interpretation involves putting collected data into the context of the program or service and determining whether goals were met or outcomes were accomplished. It is important to develop this section of the report to fully explain any results that indicate the program or service did not have its intended effect as well as a description of outcomes identified as a part of the evaluation that were not expected. Unanticipated outcomes or failing to meet predetermined goals can indicate that the suppositions used to develop the program were wrong. They can also be an indication that there was a flaw in the program design. It is, therefore, important to fully describe and interpret any negative or unexpected outcomes and to identify what may have gone wrong. This will help improve the program (Grinnel & Unrae, 2008). For example, if a program relied heavily on printed handout material written in English in a program of largely non-English speakers, the program will probably not meet its goals.

6. Recommendations: These should reflect the questions asked as a part of the evaluation and the findings for each question. Recommendations provided should enable the program staff to improve the program.

USING EVALUATION RESULTS

The ultimate purpose of program evaluation is to use the information generated to improve programs. The results of an evaluation can improve organizational management and planning, assist in decision-making, and indicate where improvement is needed. Patton (2002) has noted that the use of evaluation findings does not just happen; the process must be facilitated. Some strategies to facilitate the use of findings include the following: (a) Engage stakeholders early in the preparation for the evaluation and design the evaluation to achieve intended uses by stakeholders; (b) prepare stakeholders for eventual use by rehearsing how different conclusions could affect outcomes; (c) provide continuous feedback to stakeholders as the evaluation progresses, particularly those that might affect the use of findings; (d) schedule follow-up meetings with intended users to facilitate the transfer of evaluation findings into strategic decision-making; (e) establish a monitoring mechanism to determine how well evaluation findings and recommendations are used (MacDonald et al., 2001).

CONCLUSIONS

A program evaluation is intended to continually improve a program or service. Although it is important to demonstrate how successful the program was, it is equally important to understand why some aspects of the program did not work as well as intended. Evaluation is designed to uncover all aspects of the evaluation: what worked, what didn't work, and what needs to be improved (Evaluation Toolbox, 2010).

■ QUESTIONS FOR DISCUSSION

Evaluation questions focus on evaluation and reflect the purpose of the evaluation as well as the priorities and needs of the stakeholders. Questions should be structured to provide answers to the program component you are interested in evaluating. Consider the following scenarios and develop evaluation questions for them. Are your questions process or outcome questions? What stakeholders would have to be involved to answer the questions and what resources would you need?

1. What are the facilitators and challenges to doing intake interviews in the new mental health clinic?
2. What is the efficacy of a new breast screening protocol?
3. Is everything in place so that accreditation reports can be written quickly and easily?
4. How is the installation of a new electronic health record system going?
5. How much is recidivism among heart failure patients costing us?

■ REFLECTIVE EXERCISE

Read the following article about a program evaluation. Determine how the goals were defined, how they were measured, and whether the program was successful. Discuss how the guiding principles inform the ethical practice of this evaluation.

Wolf, Z. R., & Bailey, D. N.(2018). Nursing center-health intervention program in Philadelphia: Program evaluation and outcomes. *Nursing Forum, 53*(2), 161–172. doi:10.1111/nuf.12238

EXAMPLES OF PROGRAM EVALUATION

Trying to Bridge the Worlds of Home Visitation and Child Welfare: Lessons Learned From a Formative Evaluation

Young children in families who are a part of a child welfare system are at high risk of recurrent maltreatment and poor developmental outcomes. This article describes findings from a formative evaluation of a program designed to connect child welfare–involved families to an existing evidence-supported home visitation program as a preventive resource for families. The program was developed by a service–academic partnership, including leaders from a public state child welfare system, early childhood education specialists, and agencies providing family support services. Despite extensive and rigorous planning by the workgroup and collaborative refining of the intervention approach as agency needs changed, the changes within both the home visitation agency and the child welfare agencies created significant ongoing barriers to implementation. On the other hand, child welfare–involved families were receptive to engaging with home visitation.

Reference

Stahlschmidt, M. J., Jonson-Reid, M., Pons, L., Constantino, J., Kohl, P. L., Drake, B., & Auslander, W. I. (2018). Trying to bridge the worlds of home visitation and child welfare: Lessons learned from a formative evaluation. *Evaluation and Program Planning, 66*, 133–140. doi:10.1016/j.evalprogplan.2017.10.001

Summative Evaluation of Patient Satisfaction Strategies in an Urban Emergency Department

Background: Externally conducted surveys of patient satisfaction are the norm in hospitals today and are linked to hospital reimbursement. This initiative provides an incentive to improve patient care and develop processes to improve the patient experience. A significant decrease in patient satisfaction scores was observed over a two-quarter period in a large urban emergency department (ED). This decrease in scores occurred after a lengthy process to address low patient satisfaction scores the previous year. A protocol was developed for all staff to follow, which initially resulted in a significant increase in scores. The decrease in scores prompted an evaluation as to why this was occurring.

Aim: The purpose of this study was to conduct an evaluation of the measures used initially that were instrumental in increasing patient satisfaction-related scores and to determine whether those measures are still the best strategies to use and to suggest alternative strategies as appropriate. An additional aim was to determine the ED staff's accountability for the protocol. A proxy definition of patient satisfaction was used in this project that included nurse-sensitive indicators such as the following: (a) nurse courtesy, (b) the time taken by nurses to listen, and (c) nurses being informative regarding treatment.

Method: Summative evaluation is referred to as an *ex-post evaluation* (after the event) and is associated with accountability. Direct and random

(*continued*)

EXAMPLES OF CASE STUDY PROJECTS (*CONTINUED*)

observations of staff were conducted to determine whether the protocol developed 1 year prior to increase patient satisfaction scores was still being followed. These observations were documented on a checklist designed for specific areas within the ED, such as: triage, urgent care, main ED, and waiting room. The protocol developed as a part of the initial effort to increase scores was used as the checklist for this observation. The observation was conducted at random times and on random days. The day of the observation was randomly selected from a bag containing all of the days of the week. In turn, the time of observation was selected randomly from another bag containing 1-hour time frames for observation. The staff observed were selected from among those on duty during the selected time and day using the same method. All observed staff were seen in interaction with patients while completing a full range of patient care activities in all of the ED areas.

Findings: The results of the direct observations showed variations in the adoption of the protocol by the majority of staff observed. These findings supported that the significant drop in the proxy patient satisfaction scores during the fourth quarter could have contributed to the variations and inconsistencies in using the protocol.

Conclusion: A consistent standard work guideline is necessary in order to improve the perception of care by the patients and their families. It was obvious during this evaluation that the established protocol was not being followed. The ED performance improvement committee recommended that the work protocol be further refined and introduced anew through hiring and orientation of staff and that continuing staff be held accountable for the tenets of the protocol through yearly evaluation.

Reference

Singer, A. (2011). Summative evaluation of patient satisfaction strategies in an urban emergency department. In C. Holly (Ed.), *Scholarly inquiry and the DNP capstone* (p. 171). New York, NY: Springer Publishing.

■ SUGGESTED READINGS

Bremer, E., Graham, J. D., Veldhuizen, S., & Cairney, J. A. (2018). Program evaluation of an in-school daily physical activity initiative for children and youth. *BMC Public Health, 18*(1), 1023. doi:10.1186/s12889-018-5943-2

Epstein, D., & Klerman, J. A. (2012). When is a program ready for rigorous impact evaluation? The role of a falsifiable logic model. *Evaluation Review, 36*(5), 375–401. doi:10.1177/0193841X12474275

Gill, S., Kuwahara, R., & Wilce, M. (2016). Through a culturally competent lens: Why the program evaluation standards matter. *Health Promotion Practice, 17*(1), 5–8. doi:10.1177/1524839915616364

■ REFERENCES

American Evaluation Association. (2013). Evaluation competencies has developed a set of guidelines for the design and conduct of evaluation activities. Retrieved from http://www.eval.org/GPTraining/GP%20Training%20Final/gp.principles.pdf

Beyer, B. (1995). *How to conduct a formative evaluation*. Washington, DC: Association for the Supervision of Curriculum Development. Retrieved from http://isites.harvard.edu/fs/docs/icb.topic541040.files/A_beyer1995pp1-36_44-57_66-70_78-81.pdf

Centers for Disease Control and Prevention. (2011). *Developing an effective evaluation plan*. Atlanta, GA: Centers for Disease Control and Prevention, National Center for Chronic Disease Prevention and Health Promotion, Office on Smoking and Health; Division of Nutrition, Physical Activity, and Obesity. Retrieved from http://www.cdc.gov/obesity/downloads/CDC-Evaluation-Workbook-508.pdf

Evaluation Toolbox. (2010). Retrieved from http://www.evaluationtoolbox.net.au/index.php?option=com_content&view=article&id=15&Itemid=19

Grinnel, R., & Unrae, Y. (2008). *Social work research and evaluation* (8th ed.). New York, NY: Oxford University Press.

Hendricks, M., Plantz, M. C., & Pritchard, K. J. (2008). Measuring outcomes of United Way–funded programs: Expectations and reality. In J. G. Carman & K. A. Fredericks (Eds.), *Nonprofits and evaluation. Vol. 119: New directions for evaluation* (pp. 13–35). San Francisco, CA: Jossey Bass.

Holly, C., Rittenmeyer, L., & Weeks, S. (2014). Evidence based clinical audit criteria for the prevention and management of acute delirium in the post-operative patient with a hip fracture. *Orthopedic Nursing, 33*(1), 27–34.

Jenner, E., Jenner, L.W., Matthews-Sterling, M.. Butts, J., & Evans Williams, T. (2010). Awareness effects of a youth suicide prevention media campaign in Louisiana. *Suicide and Life-Threatening Behavior, 40*(4), 394–406. doi:10.1521/suli.2010.40.4.394

Landau, V. (2001). *Developing a project management plan instructor's notes*. Retrieved from http://www.roundworldmedia.com/cvc/module10/notes10.html

MacDonald, G., Starr, G., Schooley, M., Yee, S. L., Klimowski, K., & Turner, K. (2001). *Introduction to program evaluation for comprehensive tobacco control programs*. Atlanta, GA: Centers for Disease Control and Prevention. Retrieved from http://www.cdc.gov/tobacco/tobacco_control_programs/surveillance_evaluation/evaluation_manual/pdfs/evaluation.pdf

Patton, M. Q. (2002). *Utilization-focused evaluation (U-FE) checklist*. Retrieved from http://www.mymande.org/sites/default/files/ufe.pdf

Patton, M. Q. (2008). *Utilization focused evaluation* (4th ed.). Thousand Oaks, CA: Sage.

Pennel, C. L., McLeroy, K. R., Burdine, J. N., & Matarrita-Cascante, D. A. (2015). Nonprofit hospitals' approach to community health needs assessment. *Journal of Public Health, 105*(3), e103–e113. doi:10.2105/AJPH.2014.302286

Plochg, T., Delnoij, D., van der Kruk, T., Janmaat, T., & Klazinga, N. (2005). Intermediate care: For better or worse? Process evaluation of an intermediate care model between a university hospital and a residential home. *BMC Health Services Research, 5*, 38. doi:10.1186/1472-6963-5-38

Rossi, P., Lipsey, M., & Freeman, H. (2004). *Evaluation: A systematic approach* (7th ed.). Thousand Oaks, CA: Sage.

Stetler, C. B., Legro, M. W., Wallace, C. M., Bowman, C., Guihan, M., Hagedorn, H., . . . Smith, J. L. (2006). The role of formative evaluation in implementation research and the QUERI experience. *Journal of General Internal Medicine, 21*, S1–S8. doi:10.1007/s11606-006-0267-9

CHAPTER 13

Descriptive Observational Projects

OBJECTIVES

At the end of this chapter, you will be able to:

- Differentiate among the types of descriptive observational projects.
- Explain the various types of bias and confounding variables found in descriptive observational projects.
- Understand the concept of significance.
- Select a descriptive observational project design to answer a practice question.

KEY CONCEPTS

- A descriptive observational project involves observing without influencing or interfering with behavior.
- Although the randomized controlled trial (RCT) is considered the gold standard and principal design for evaluation of interventions, procedures, and services, there are many aspects of care that cannot be tested or evaluated in a randomized fashion.

INTRODUCTION

A descriptive doctor of nursing practice (DNP) project is about observations. An observation is a description of a phenomenon. Observations can be qualitative (watching) or quantitative (a laboratory test).

© Springer Publishing Company DOI: 10.1891/9780826134943.0013

This type of project can be a descriptive observational project (prevalence surveys, case series, case reports) or an analytical observational project (cohort, case control, cross-sectional). Qualitative descriptive projects are discussed in Chapter 7. The investigator's role in these studies is to observe, record, and analyze results and make inferences based on the findings; the investigator does not intervene or manipulate. See Table 13.1 for a further description of these approaches.

Observational projects are designed to answer questions about a naturally occurring phenomenon. For example, Alsulami, Choonara, and Conroy (2014) observed pediatric nurses' adherence to double-checking during medication administration; 2,000 medication dose administration events were observed. They found that drug dose calculation, rate of administering intravenous bolus drugs, and labeling of flush syringes had the lowest adherence rates. Drug dose calculation was only double-checked in 591 (30%) of the 2,000 drug administrations. Medication administration errors ($n = 191$) or deviations from policy were observed at a rate of 9.6% of drug administrations. These included 64 drug doses that were left for parents to administer without nurse observation.

DESCRIPTIVE AND ANALYTIC OBSERVATIONAL STUDIES

Observational studies can be either descriptive or analytic. Descriptive studies examine the frequency of occurrence and analytic studies evaluate the relationships among different exposures. Descriptive studies include case series/case reports and prevalence surveys, whereas analytic studies include cohort studies, case-control studies, and cross-sectional studies.

The most common observational study is the descriptive study. Descriptive studies are observational studies that describe patterns related to person, place, and time; they do not establish cause and effect. Descriptive studies do not have a comparison (control) group, which means that they do not allow for inferences to be drawn about associations (Heffernan, 2010). For example, Aznar et al. (2010) studied patterns of physical activity in Spanish children. Their findings indicated that few children achieved the exercise levels recommended for health; at greatest risk were adolescent girls.

Descriptive study designs include case reports, case series, incidence studies, and ecologic studies. The case report follows the most basic design. It is a story about something that happened in a medical setting, such as an adverse reaction to medication or an unexpected event, such as a fall with injuries. The case series design is an extension

TABLE 13.1

RESEARCH DESIGNS FOR OBSERVATIONAL STUDIES

Study Design	Description	Data Collection	Advantages	Disadvantages
Prospective cohort study	A longitudinal study of a group of people who share a common characteristic, such as year of high school graduation or taking the same drug	Medical records Environmental or lifestyle questionnaires Physiological measurement Interview data	Allows investigation of rare diseases or diseases with a long latency Can measure risk Large cohorts can minimize selection bias Aides in understanding causal associations Can test hypotheses	Subjects are not randomly assigned High attrition rates Expensive to conduct Long time to obtain useful data for analysis
Retrospective cohort studies	A historical study of a group of people who share a common characteristic, such as smoking and heart disease or working in a coal mine	Medical records	Less expensive and faster than a prospective cohort study Can test hypotheses	Lack of follow-up affects study validity

(continued)

TABLE 13.1 (CONTINUED)

RESEARCH DESIGNS FOR OBSERVATIONAL STUDIES

Study Design	Description	Data Collection	Advantages	Disadvantages
Case-control studies	A study of "cases" who have a condition or exposure in comparison with "controls," cases who do not have the condition or exposure	Medical records Registry data Death certificates Population surveys	Allows understanding of risk factors Inexpensive Few personnel needed Useful for studying outcomes that take a long time to develop, for example, cancer Can test hypotheses	There is a better recall of information among exposed groups (recall bias) Odds ratios are used as a proxy measure for relative risk
Case series/case report	A tracking study of people given a similar treatment, such as the use of an automated external defibrillator for out-of-hospital cardiac arrest survival	Medical records Detailed patient reports	Adverse events and side effects are identified Can generate hypotheses	

Cross-sectional studies	A descriptive study of a group of people at one point in time, a "snapshot"; also called a *prevalence study*	Survey methods Secondary data	Provides a foundation for the stronger cohort or RCT designs Can generate hypotheses	No control group Difficult to determine when the outcome of interest began, as everything is measured at one time
Descriptive studies	Descriptive studies identify descriptive characteristics; they are an important first step in the search for determinants or risk factors that can be altered or eliminated to reduce or prevent disease		Hypothesis generating Can be useful in establishing trends or patterns	

RCT, randomized control trial.

of the case report in which several events are described. These events usually have been observed over time in one setting. This study can be retrospective or prospective. For example, Lovell, Bajwah, Maddocks, Wilcock, and Higginson (2018) reviewed six cases in which mirtazapine, an antidepressant, was used to treat chronic breathlessness in advanced lung disease. All cases received mirtazapine at a starting dose of 15 mg. All cases reported less breathlessness and being more active. Patients described feeling more in control of their breathing and being able to recover more quickly from episodes of breathlessness. Some cases also reported beneficial effects on anxiety, panic, appetite, and sleep. No adverse effects were reported.

Analytic observational studies are designed to address a specific research hypothesis, usually about the effect of an exposure on an outcome. Analytic studies use either group or individual data, except for ecologic studies, in which only group data are used. An ecologic study is an examination of risk-modifying factors on health or other outcomes in a geographically or temporally defined population. Sanders et al. (2014) investigated the association between metal concentrations (arsenic, cadmium, manganese, lead) in private wells and birth defects. Using registry data, the study consisted of 20,151 infants born with selected birth defects (cases) and 668,381 nonmalformed infants (controls). Maternal residences at delivery and over 10,000 well locations measured for metals were geocoded. Elevated manganese levels were statistically significantly associated with a higher prevalence of conotruncal heart defects, that is, tetralogy of Fallot, pulmonary atresia with ventricular septal defect (prevalence ratio [PR]: 1.6, 95% confidence interval [CI]: 1.1–2.5).These findings suggest an ecologic association between higher manganese concentrations in drinking water and the prevalence of conotruncal heart defects.

A cohort study is a longitudinal observational study whose focus is on exposure or risk. A cohort study has a control group. The group is followed over time to examine an outcome of interest and map its long-term effects, as in the Framingham Heart Study (FHS). The FHS has followed three generations of participants for over 70 years to identify the common factors or characteristics that contribute to cardiovascular disease (CVD; www.framinghamheartstudy.org). In other words, a cohort study starts with cohorts of well individuals and follows them until events occur. Chen et al. (2015) investigated the risks between peripheral artery disease (PAD) and carbon monoxide (CO) poisoning. This population-based cohort study analyzed registry data from 1998 to 2010 with a follow-up period to the end of 2011. In this study, 9,046 patients with CO poisoning and 36,183 controls were included. The overall risks for developing PAD were 1.85-fold in the patients with CO poisoning compared with the comparison cohort after adjusting for age, gender, and comorbidities. Long-term cohort study results showed a higher risk for PAD development among patients with CO poisoning.

A case-control study is an observational study with a control group. A particular disease or condition is the starting point—the case—and the study investigates in a backward (retrospective) fashion to determine a cause and any associated risk factors. The cases are known and they exhibit symptoms of the condition under study that might be expected. Controls must be similar to the cases, except that that they do not have the outcome in question (Holly, Salmond, & Saimbert, 2016). For example, Suarez et al. (2010) used a multistate registry on birth defects to examine the relation between neural tube defects and maternal exposure to cigarette smoke. Results indicated that compared with nonsmokers, mothers exposed only to passive smoke had an increased neural tube defect odds ratio (*OR*: 1.7, 95% CI: 1.4–2.0), adjusted for race, ethnicity, and study center, suggesting that maternal exposure to passive smoking increases the incidence of neural tube defects in infants.

A cross-sectional study is a descriptive study that gathers information on both the condition and the exposure at the same time. Cross-sectional studies provide a "snapshot" of one point in time. This type of data can be used to assess the prevalence of acute or chronic conditions in a population. A cross-sectional study is sometimes called a *prevalence study*.

SIGNIFICANCE IN OBSERVATIONAL STUDIES

Significance refers to the probability that a relationship could be caused by chance. Either a *p* value or a CI is used to determine whether results are statistically significant. When statistical significance is expressed in terms of a *p* value, the *p* refers to *probability*. A *p* value of less than .05, which is the usual value used in doctor of nursing practice (DNP) projects, implies there is a less than one in 20, or five in 100, chance of something happening. When *p* values are this small, the results of the study are interpreted to be significant; that is, it is unlikely to have resulted through chance. A *p* value at the level of .01 is considered to be "highly significant." *P* values this small indicate that the results could occur less than once in 100 times (Crombie & Davies, 2003).

CIs can also be used to determine the significance of study results. A CI is the range of values that encompass a population parameter. Because it is impossible to measure a total population, the study sample is used to calculate a range in which population value will most likely fall. This is known as the *95% CI*. A 95% CI is a range of values that you can be 95% certain contain the true mean of the population. The values at either end of the range are known as the *confidence limits*; the wider the CI, the less accurate it is (Crombie & Davies, 2003). CIs are sensitive to variability in the population (spread of values) and sample size. When used to compare the means of two or more treatment groups, a CI shows the magnitude of a difference between groups.

The two definitions of statistical significance are compatible. If you have a *p* value of less than .05, it is the same as getting a 95% CI that does not overlap zero. In the reverse, a *p* value greater than .05 equates to a 95% CI, which includes 1 (the null value), meaning that there is no effect (Crombie & Davies, 2003).

BIAS AND CONFOUNDING IN OBSERVATIONAL STUDIES

An observational study has the potential to provide results that may prove misleading due to confounding factors, biases, or both. In an observational study, bias is a deviation of a measurement from the truth, leading to either an underestimation or overestimation of significance, and can be related to the way in which the study was designed, conducted, or interpreted. Bias may result from poor diagnosis or poor diagnostic criteria, poor case choice, poor choice of controls, or variation in the way data were collected or measured. The internal validity of the study is affected by any bias present (Jepsen, Johnsen, Gillma, & Sorensen, 2004).

Two potential biases that may limit the suitability of an observational study are selection bias and information bias (Jepsen et al., 2004). Box 13.1 presents questions to ask to determine whether a bias is present in an observational study. Selection bias means that the sample is not representative of the population. Selection bias is more common in case-control studies than in cohort studies. Examples of selection bias include self-selection, volunteerism, attrition, and lack of follow-up (Jepsen et al., 2004).

Information bias, also known as *classification* or *measurement bias*, refers to an error in measuring the exposure or outcome, usually in a cohort study. Information bias can occur in a variety of ways, including differences in the way information is gathered (in person vs. telephone), coded, entered, or interpreted. For example, an interviewer may transcribe information inaccurately. In case-control studies that rely on memory of past experiences, information bias is referred to as *recall bias*, meaning those in the exposed group may have better recall or better information than the healthier controls (Grimes & Schultz, 2002; Jepsen et al., 2004; Table 13.2).

BOX 13.1

QUESTIONS TO ASK TO DETERMINE BIAS IN OBSERVATIONAL RESEARCH

1. To determine whether a selection bias is present, ask:
   In a cohort study, are participants in the exposed and unexposed groups alike in all key aspects except for the exposure?
   In a case-control study, are cases and controls alike in all key aspects except for the condition under study?
2. To determine whether an information bias is present, ask:
   In a cohort study, is information about outcome obtained in exactly the same way for both exposed and unexposed groups?
   In a case-control study, is information about exposure collected in the same way for cases and controls?
3. To determine whether a confounding is present, ask:
   Could the results be accounted for by the presence of a factor that was not considered a priori, for example, smoking, diet, or activity level?

Source: Grimes, D. A., & Schultz, K. F. (2002). Bias and causal relationships in observational research. *Lancet, 359,* 248–252. doi:10.1016/S0140-6736(02)07451-2

TABLE 13.2

TYPES OF BIAS

Type of Bias	Explanation of Bias	Critical Appraisal for Bias
Selection bias	• Definition: Results from errors in the way that research participants were selected into the study from the target population or as a result of factors that influence whether research participants remained in a study. • The intervention group is different from the control/comparison group in baseline characteristics. • The participants are not representative of the population of all possible participants. • Nonrandom samples are at greatest risk for selection bias.	Randomization and allocation concealment are key to minimizing selection bias. Evaluate whether: • Randomization was used. • The allocation sequence was appropriate and adequately concealed.

(continued)

TABLE 13.2 (CONTINUED)

TYPES OF BIAS		
Type of Bias	Explanation of Bias	Critical Appraisal for Bias
Performance bias	• Definition: Systematic differences exist in care provided to the participants in the intervention and control/comparison group. • This bias is more likely to occur if the caregiver is aware of whether a patient is in a control or treatment group.	Was there blinding of the subject? Was there blinding of the researcher/ clinician?
Attrition bias	• Definition: Differences exist between control and treatment groups in terms of patients dropping out of a study or not being followed. • Although dropouts will occur, investigators want to be assured that missing outcome data are balanced in numbers across groups with similar reasons for missing data across groups.	Was loss to follow-up (dropout, nonresponse, withdrawal, protocol deviators) reported? Did researchers apply the concept of intention to treat?
Detection (assessor or ascertainment) bias	• Definition: Occurs if outcomes are measured differently for patients depending on whether they are in the control or treatment group. • A detection bias generally occurs when the assessor (the one determining the outcome results) knows whether the subject is in the control or intervention group.	Was blinding of the assessor carried out?

Source: Holly, C., Salmond, S., & Saimbert, M. (2016). *Comprehensive systematic review for advanced nursing practice*. New York: Sage.

A *confounding* is a clouding of resultgs Institutes such that the outcomes of a study cannot be clearly determined. Although bias involves error in the measurement of a variable, confounding involves error in the interpretation of the measurement (Joanna Briggs Institute, 2008). For example, lung cancer (outcome) is less common in people with asthma (variable). However, it is improbable that asthma provides protection against lung cancer. It is more likely that the occurrence of lung cancer is lower in people with asthma because fewer asthmatics smoke cigarettes (confounding variable; Mann, 2003).

CONCLUSIONS

A descriptive observational study is a common type of study in which the investigator passively observes, rather than intervenes. The two most common are:

- Descriptive observational studies, which collect information on the distribution of disease patterns in terms of the characteristics of person, place, and time.
- Analytical observational studies, which test a causal hypothesis concerning the relationship between exposure and disease. These include the cohort and case-control studies.

This type of design can be used in a DNP project to collect baseline data for an intervention study or determine the prevalence of a condition (e.g., hospital-acquired pressure ulcers) so that an intervention can be implemented.

■ QUESTION FOR DISCUSSION

You have decided to do a project involving training in disaster preparedness in a hospital system using a survey. Describe what you can do to make the survey as representative as possible.

■ REFLECTIVE EXERCISE

Think about a practice problem you have recently encountered, for example, an increase in fall rates or increased rates of physical restraint use.

1. Use the PICO (patient, intervention, comparison, outcome) method to study this problem, listing each of the four considerations.
2. Rewrite the PICO as a research question.
3. What type of research design would you use to study this problem?

4. What sampling strategy would you use?
5. What data would you collect and how would you analyze them?

EXAMPLE OF AN OBSERVATIONAL STUDY

Breastfeeding and the Weekend Effect: An Observational Study
This study compared the incidence of breastfeeding by day of week of birth using a retrospective database of 16,508 records from the Infant Feeding Survey in the United Kingdom. Among babies of mothers who left full-time education aged 16 or under, the incidence of breastfeeding was 6.7 percentage points lower (95% CI: 1.4,12.1) for those born on Saturdays than for those born on Mondays–Thursdays. No such differences by day of week of birth were observed among babies of mothers who left school aged 17 or over.

Reference
Fitzsimons, E., & Vera-Hernández, M. (2016). Breast feeding and the weekend effect: An observational study. *BMJ Open, 6*(7), e010016. doi:10.1136/bmjopen-2015-010016

■ SUGGESTED READINGS

O'Brien, S. F., & Yi, Q. (2016). How do I interpret a confidence interval? *Transfusion, 56*(7), 1680–1683. doi:10.1111/trf.13635

Toledano, M. B., Smith, R. B., Brook, J. P., Douglass, M., & Elliott, P. (2015). How to establish and follow up a large prospective cohort study in the 21st century—Lessons from UK COSMOS. *PLoS One, 10*(7), e0131521. doi:10.1371/journal.pone.0131521

■ REFERENCES

Alsulami, Z., Choonara, I., & Conroy, S. (2014). Paediatric nurses' adherence to the double-checking process during medication administration in a children's hospital: An observational study. *Journal of Advanced Nursing, 70*(6), 1404–1413. doi:10.1111/jan.12303

Aznar, S., Naylor, P. J., Silva, P., Pérez, M., Angulo, T., Laguna, M., . . . López-Chicharro, J. (2010). Patterns of physical activity in Spanish children: A descriptive pilot study. *Child: Care, Health and Development.* Epub ahead of print November 18. doi:10.1111/j.1365-2214.2010.01175.x

Chen, Y. G., Lin, T. Y., Dai, M. S., Lin, C. L., Hung, Y., Huang, W. S., & Kao, C. H. (2015). Risk of peripheral artery disease in patients with carbon monoxide poisoning: A population-based retrospective cohort study. *Medicine, 94*(40), e1608. doi:10.1097/MD.0000000000001608

Crombie, I., & Davies, H. (2003). *What is meta-analysis.* London, UK: Hayward Medical Communications.

Fitzsimons, E., & Vera-Hernández, M. (2016). Breast feeding and the weekend effect: An observational study. *BMJ Open, 6*(7), e010016. doi:10.1136/bmjopen-2015-010016

Grimes, D. A., & Schultz, K. F. (2002). Bias and causal relationships in observational research. *Lancet, 359*, 248–252. doi:10.1016/S0140-6736(02)07451-2

Heffernan, C. (2010). *Ask Dr. Cath*. Retrieved from http://www.drcath.net/index.html

Holly, C., Salmond, S., & Saimbert, M. (2016). *Comprehensive systematic review for advanced nursing practice*. New York, NY: Sage.

Jepsen, P., Johnsen, S. P., Gillma, M. W., & Sorensen, H. T. (2004). Interpretation of observational studies. *Heart, 90*(8), 956–960. doi:10.1136/hrt.2003.017269

Joanna Briggs Institute. (2008). *Reviewers manual*. Adelaide, AU: University of Adelaide.

Leeflang, M. M., Deeks, J. J., Takwoingi, Y., & Macaskill, P. (2013). Cochrane diagnostic test accuracy reviews. *Systematic Reviews, 2*, 82. doi:10.1186/2046-4053-2-82

Lovell, N., Bajwah, S., Maddocks, M., Wilcock, A., & Higginson, I. J. (2018). Use of mirtazapine in patients with chronic breathlessness: A case series. *Palliative Medicine, 32*(9), 1518–1521. doi:10.1177/0269216318787450

Mann, C. (2003). Observational research methods. *Emergency Medicine Journal, 20*(1), 54–60. doi:10.1136/emj.20.1.54

Sanders, A. P., Desrosiers, T. A., Warren, J. L., Herring, A. H., Enright, D., Olshan, A. F., . . . Fry, R. C. (2014). Association between arsenic, cadmium, manganese, and lead levels in private wells and birth defects prevalence in North Carolina: A semi-ecologic study. *BMC Public Health, 14*, 955. doi:10.1186/1471-2458-14-955

CHAPTER 14

Disseminating the Results of the DNP Project

▨ OBJECTIVES

At the end of the chapter, you will be able to:

- Explain the importance of disseminating project findings.
- Identify ways to disseminate the results of the DNP project.

▨ KEY CONCEPTS

- The last step in the project process is dissemination of findings—allowing project findings to become part of the body of knowledge about a topic.
- Disseminating knowledge is critical for any discipline.
- Dissemination of a DNP project is necessary to enhance and further nursing practice.

INTRODUCTION

The DNP project is a unique opportunity to advance nursing art and science, but only if the information is presented beyond the university where the degree was obtained (Stoner, 2018). Clarke and Garcia (2015) note that it is critical for nurses to have access to the most current thinking in their field and this can only occur if findings of DNP projects are disseminated. Although dissemination of DNP project findings may be the hardest step in the process, there are several reasons to disseminate outcomes:

- Disseminating knowledge gained through clinically focused projects is essential for advancing a practice discipline.
- Disseminating results establishes expertise in a specific clinical area.
- Without disseminating results, no one will be able to benefit from the findings.
- Dissemination may contribute to career goals in some places of employment. Publication and presentation have long been required in academia and increasingly in service agencies.
- The emphasis on dissemination is a common requirement of advancement at a Magnet hospital.

Dissemination involves spreading information to people who can most benefit from knowing the information. For decades, this meant publishing articles in professional journals following specific author guidelines. Recently, dissemination of findings has taken different forms (Table 14.1). The traditional journal publication is no longer emphasized by the American Association of Colleges of Nursing (AACN) for DNP programs. Rather, AACN has specified that DNP programs should focus on the translation of new science and its application and evaluation.

TABLE 14.1

DISSEMINATING DNP PROJECT OUTCOMES

Type	Example
Print	Peer-reviewed journal Review of the literature based on the project Letters to the editor Policy briefs for elected representatives
Presentation	Podium or poster presentations at conferences Continuing-education sessions
Digita Imedia	YouTube Twitter Facebook Personal website Blogs Podcasts

DNP, doctor of nursing practice.

Source: Stoner, M. (2018). *A guide to disseminating your DNP project.* New York, NY: Springer Publishing.

Graduates of DNP programs should be able to generate new knowledge, translate evidence, and implement evidence using quality-improvement processes in specific practice settings or systems or with specific populations to improve health or health outcomes (AACN, 2015).

PUBLISHING IN A JOURNAL

Publishing in a peer-reviewed journal can be the most effective method of sharing findings with a large group of clinicians or researchers. Articles can be published online or in print. Some things to remember when considering publishing some or all of a project's findings in a nursing journal:

- When you submit your article, select a clinical journal in a specialty area that relates to your topic. A comprehensive, alphabetized list of nursing journals can be found on the website of the International Academy of Nursing Editors (nursingeditors.com).
- Do not send the entire DNP capstone report to the journal. You need to be sure to follow the journal's author guidelines. These guidelines are available on the journal website. There are page, word, and style guidelines that must be followed.
- Because you can submit a manuscript to only one journal at a time, choose the one with the best fit for your work. Submitting a manuscript to more than one journal at a time is construed as ethical misconduct. To be sure that you are following ethical guidelines for publication, consult the COPE (Council on Publication Ethics) website (www.cope.org).
- Establish a writing routine. Try to set aside a regular time for scholarly writing; 15 minutes a day in an area where there are minimal distractions will allow you to complete your work quickly.
- Find the right writing tools. The most important tool is a word-processing application, such as Microsoft Word. You want to be able to write and maneuver through documents quickly, cutting and pasting, moving text, changing from portrait to landscape, finding and replacing words, merging documents, creating bulleted lists or tables, inserting symbols, and so on. Take advantage of the free tutorial online at GCFLearnFree.org. Teach yourself to use EndNote (from Thomson Reuters) or RefWorks (from ProQuest) if you did not do so as part of your DNP project. These programs save and organize articles and format your reference list (Roush, 2017).

■ Review the author guidelines carefully. These provide guidance for submitting work to the journal based on the article type. Some journals may require that you follow specific guidelines based on the type of article you are submitting. Some of these may be:

CONSORT (Consolidated Standards of Reporting Trials): www.consort-statement.org
PRISMA (Preferred Reporting Items for Systematic Reviews and Meta-Analyses): www.prisma-statement.org
SQUIRE (Standards for Quality Improvement Reporting Excellence): www.squire-statement.org
TREND (Transparent Reporting of Evaluations with Nonrandomized Designs): www.cdc.gov/trendstatement

■ Know the style followed by the journal. Two of the most common styles are APA, named for the American Psychological Association (www.apastyle.org) and MLA named for the Modern Language Association of America(www.mla.org).
■ Before you send in your article, get feedback on what you have written from colleagues who have published articles.

Before you begin, consider taking the free online course "Writing for Professional Journals" open to the public and licensed under Creative Commons (nursing.utah.edu/journalwriting).

CONFERENCE PRESENTATION

Choosing a conference at which to make a presentation can be a similar process to choosing a journal. Look for conferences that align with objectives that relate to your project. It is necessary to submit an for the conference planners to determine the fit of your project with their conference objectives. When you submit an abstract to a conference, you can opt to present your work in a poster, an oral paper, or either and leave it up to the conference committee to decide (Roush, 2017).

An abstract is a short, stand-alone summary of the entire project. It describes the background, purpose, method, results, and conclusions of the project. A committee of clinical experts reviews each abstract to decide which best meet the objectives of a conference and are worthy of presentation. The following should be included in an abstract:

- Background: Include one to two sentences on the background of the article. For example, use the background statement: *Cognitive impairment is a recognized predictor of acute delirium, particularly in the postoperative period.*
- Problem Statement/Purpose: Include one to two sentences about the purpose and scope of the article. For example, *The purpose of this article is to describe the occurrence of cognitive impairment in postoperative surgical patients as a predictor of acute delirium.*
- Method/Approach: Add two to three sentences on how you conducted the project. What variables were included or excluded? For example, *A medical record review of 1,200 patients admitted to a large urban hospital was conducted.*
- Results/Findings: Include two to three sentences on what you found. Was the question answered or the purpose met? For example, *Cognitive impairment was second only to age as the most common predictor of delirium in postoperative patients.*
- Conclusions/Implications: Allow two to three sentences detailing the importance of your findings. Are the results generalizable? For example, *To decrease the incidence of delirium and to keep patients safe, maintain their functionality, or plan for safe discharge to their original place of residence, all older adults admitted for surgical procedures should be assessed for cognitive impairment.*
- Keywords: Keywords are a list of three to five words or short phrases that describe your project. Be sure all of these words appear in the abstract. For example, *acute delirium, cognitive impairment, postoperative patients.*

If your abstract is accepted for oral presentation at a conference, you will have 10 to 20 minutes to present your project followed by a 5-minute question-and-answer period. Your presentation will most likely be a part of a session of four to five similar presentations. A PowerPoint presentation is the most common presentation method. When using a PowerPoint, limit the content on the slides to the important points, such as (Roush, 2017):

What was the question that guided the project?
Why was it an important question (background/significance)?
How do you go about answering it (method)?
What did you find out (results)?

What are the implications for practice and education?
What further questions are raised from this work?

A poster is also a way to begin disseminating project findings. Submission of an abstract for a poster presentation is appropriate for projects with a small sample size, pilot projects, projects developing evidence-based guidelines, or preliminary findings.

A poster session is about 1 to 2 hours long, during which time you must be at your poster, and conference attendees use that time to view and discuss the work presented.

CONCLUSIONS

Dissemination of the findings of a DNP project is a professional responsibility. Sharing the knowledge gained from completing a DNP project with other nurses, interdisciplinary colleagues, policy makers, and the public through print media and oral presentations is essential for the advancement of nursing science.

■ QUESTIONS FOR DISCUSSION

1. Review the characteristics of predatory journals (www. enago.com/academy/identifying-predatory-journals-using -evidence-based-characteristics). Discuss why it is not a good idea to publish in a predatory journal.

2. Watch the YouTube presentation on publication ethics by Dr. Charon Pierson (editor-in-chief of the *Journal of the American Academy of Nurse Practitioners*). This video series discusses guidelines for authors, students, and researchers on how to manage authorship, plagiarism, conflicts of interest, and retractions in the literature. Discuss how you would address these ethical issues.

3. When searching the literature for background articles for your DNP project, you find two very similar articles in two different journals. You suspect that they are the same article with a different title and the authors are the same in each article but listed in a different order. You wonder whether this is a duplicate publication, self-plagiarism, or a copyright issue. What would you do?

■ REFLECTIVE EXERCISE

Think about establishing a writing routine. Fill in the following to reflect on how you will accomplish this:

The best time for me to write is_____.

The best place for me to write is _____.

The tools I need to become more familiar with are _____.

So that I am not distracted during my writing time, I need to _____.

■ SUGGESTED READINGS

Beall's list of predatory journals and publishers. (2017). Retrieved from http://beallslist. weebly.com

Narayanaswami, P., Gronseth, G., Dubinsky, R., Penfold-Murray, R., Cox, J., Bever, C., Jr., . . . Getchius, T. S. (2015). The impact of social media on dissemination and implementation of clinical practice guidelines: A longitudinal observational study. *Journal of Medical Internet Research, 17*(8), e193. doi:10.2196/jmir.4414

Resnick, B. (2014). Dissemination of research findings: There are NO bad studies and NO negative findings. *Geriatric Nursing, 35*(2 Suppl.), S1–S2. doi:10.1016/j.gerinurse.2014.02.012

Yancey, N. R. (2016) The challenge of writing for publication: implications for teaching-learning nursing. *Nursing Science Quarterly, 29*(4), 277–282. doi:10.1177/0894318416 662931

■ REFERENCES

American Association of Colleges of Nursing. (2015). *The doctor of nursing practice: Current issues and clarifying recommendations.* Retrieved from http://www.aacnnursing. org/Portals/42/DNP/DNP-Implementation.pdf?ver=2017-08-01-105830-517

Clarke, P. N., & Garcia, J. (2015). Evolution of nursing science: Is Open Access the answer? *Nursing Science Quarterly, 28*, 284–287. doi:10.1177/0894318415599226

Roush, K. (2017). Becoming a published writer AJN. *American Journal of Nursing, 117*(3), 63–66. doi:10.1097/01.NAJ.0000513291.04075.82

Stoner, M. (2018). *A guide to disseminating your DNP project.* New York, NY: Springer Publishing.

Selected Text Resources for Practice-Based Scholarly Inquiry

ACTION RESEARCH

Herr, K., & Anderson, G. (2005). *The action research dissertation: A guide for students and faculty*. Thousand Oaks, CA: Sage.

Stringer, E. (2013). *Action research* (4th ed.). Thousand Oaks, CA: Sage.

CASE STUDY

Yin, R. (2017). *Case study research: Design and methods* (6th ed.). Thousand Oaks, CA: Sage.

CLINICAL INTERVENTION RESEARCH

Melnyk, B., & Morrison-Beedy, D. (2012). *Interventional research: Designing, conducting, analyzing, funding*. New York, NY: Springer Publishing.

CRITICAL APPRAISAL

Bootland, D., Galloway, R., S., & McWhirter, E. (2017). *Critical appraisal from papers to patient: A practical guide*. Boca Raton, FL: Taylor and Francis.

DESCRIPTIVE STUDIES

Hackshaw, A. (2015). *A concise guide to observational studies in healthcare*. Hoboken, NJ: JohnWiley & Sons.

INTEGRATIVE REVIEW

Garrard, J. (2011). *Health science literature review made easy: The matrix method.* Burlington, MA: Jones &Barlett.

PROGRAM EVALUATION

Brosanan, C., & Hickey, J. (2012). *Evaluation of health care quality in advanced practice nursing.* New York, NY: Springer Publishing.

David Royse, D., Bruce A., & Thyer, B. A. (2015). *Program evaluation: An introduction to an evidence-based approach.* Boston, MA: Cengage Learning.

QUALITATIVE DESCRIPTIVE

Saldana, J. (2013). *The coding manual for qualitative researchers.* Thousand Oaks, CA: Sage.

Sandelowski, M., & Barroso, J. (2007). *Handbook for synthesizing qualitative research.* New York, NY: Springer Publishing.

QUALITY IMPROVEMENT

Graban, M. (2016). *Lean hospitals: Improving quality, patient satisfaction and employee engagement* (3rd ed.). Boca Raton, FL: CRC Press.

Shaw, P. (2016). *Quality and performance improvement in healthcare: Theory, practice, and management* (6th ed.). Chicago, IL: AHIMA. Retrieved from www.ahima.org

SYSTEMATIC REVIEW

Cumming, G. (2012). *Understanding the statistics: Effect size, confidence intervals and meta-analysis.* New York, NY: Routledge, Francis and Taylor Group.

Holly, C., Salmond, S., & Saimbert, M. (2016). *Comprehensive systematic review for advanced nursing practice* (2nd ed.). New York, NY: Springer Publishing.

Human Subject Protection

THE BELMONT REPORT

www.hhs.gov/ohrp/regulations-and-policy/belmont-report/index.html

ELEMENTS OF A CONSENT FORM

www.hhs.gov/ohrp/regulations-and-policy/guidance/checklists/index
.html

HUMAN SUBJECT PROTECTION TRAINING

Collaborative Institutional Training Initiative (CITI): https://www.citi-
program.org/default.asp?language=english
National Institutes of Health (NIH): phrp.nihtraining.com/users/
login.php

OFFICE OF HUMAN SUBJECT PROTECTION

www.hhs.gov/ohrp

© Springer Publishing Company DOI: 10.1891/9780826134943.ap02

PRINCIPLES OF ETHICAL RESEARCH

www.apa.org/monitor/jan03/principles.aspx

TIPS FOR WRITING AN INSTITUTIONAL REVIEW BOARD APPLICATION

mindlesseating.org/pdf/IRB_Applications.doc

Selected How-To Sources for Practice-Based Inquiry

HOW TO ANALYZE DATA

Quantitative Data

CONFIDENCE INTERVALS

www.health.ny.gov/diseases/chronic/confint.htm

www.nottingham.ac.uk/nursing/sonet/rlos/ebp/confidence_intervals/index.html

STATISTICS CALCULATOR

www.graphpad.com/quickcalcs/index.cfm

STATISTICAL TESTS

statisticalhelp.com

Qualitative Data

learningstore.uwex.edu/assets/pdfs/G3658-12.PDF

HOW TO CHOOSE THE RIGHT PROJECT METHOD

hsl.lib.umn.edu/biomed/help/understanding-research-study-designs

libguides.usc.edu/content.php?pid=83009&sid=818072

www.vadscorner.com/internet7.html

HOW TO CRITICALLY APPRAISE THE LITERATURE

Centre for Evidence-Based Medicine's Tools for Critically Appraising the Evidence: tinyurl.com/pkfm8xv

Consolidated Standards of Reporting Trials (CONSORT): www.consort-statement.org

Critical Appraisal Skills Programme (CASP): www.casp-uk.net/#!aboutus/c4nz

Downs and Black Quality Checklist for Healthcare Intervention Studies: www.nccmt.ca/resources/search/9

Joanna Briggs Institute (JBI) Critical Appraisal Tools: http://joannabriggs.org/

Pragmatic-Explanatory Continuum Indicator Summary (PRECIS) framework for evaluating pragmatic and explanatory clinical trials: www.cmtpnet.org/resource-center/view/pragmatic-explanatory-continuum-indicator-summary

HOW TO DO A NEEDS ASSESSMENT TO IDENTIFY A CLINICAL PROBLEM

www.shrm.org/resourcesandtools/tools-and-samples/how-to-guides/pages/conduct-training-needs-assessment.aspx

www.ies.ncsu.edu/blog/how-to-conduct-needs-assessment-part-1-what-is-it-and-why-do-it

HOW TO EVALUATE EVIDENCE

www.hsl.unc.edu/Services/Tutorials/EBM/Evidence.htm

HOW TO KNOW YOU ARE ON THE RIGHT TRACK

Examples of Clinical Projects

https://www.doctorsofnursingpractice.org/

HOW TO SEARCH THE LITERATURE

www.hsl.unc.edu/Services/Tutorials/EBM/Question.htm

https://support.google.com/websearch/answer/134479?hl=en&ref_topic
=3081620&vid=0-635802591522179323-4179845653

HOW TO WRITE A CAPSTONE/RESEARCH PROPOSAL

researchproposalguide.com
www.design.umn.edu/current_students/info/documents/AGuideto
WritingaCapstoneProposal-CDES.pdf
www.apastyle.org/learn/tutorials/basics-tutorial.aspx

HOW TO WRITE A CLINICAL/RESEARCH QUESTION

www.hsl.unc.edu/Services/Tutorials/EBM/Question.htm
writingcenter.gmu.edu/?p=307

HOW TO WRITE A LITERATURE REVIEW

Grant, M. J., & Booth, A. (2009). A typology of reviews: An analysis of 14 review types and associated methodologies. *Health Information and Libraries Journal, 26*(2), 91–108. doi:10.1111/j.1471-1842.2009.00848.x
Language Center, Asian Institute of Technology. (2005, February 17). Writing a literature review. Retrieved from: http://web.pdx.edu/~bertini/pdf/literature_review.pdf
OWL at Purdue University. (2003). Sample APA papers: Literature review. Retrieved from: https://library.ithaca.edu/sp/assets/users/_lch-abot/sample_apa_style_litreview.pdf
library.usm.maine.edu/tutorials/esp/module3/21_write.htm

HOW TO WRITE THE FINAL REPORT

writingcenter.unc.edu/handouts/dissertations

Index